THE DAIRY-FREE & GLUTEN-FREE COOKBOOK

100+ BASIC AND FULFILLING RECIPES WITHOUT DAIRY OR GLUTEN

By

CHLOE H. OSORIO

Table of Contents

Introduction

Rather than zeroing in on what you can't eat now, why not consider all the extraordinary food that you can eat and praise the way that you can in any case eat your number one feasts they will simply have a marginally various fixings in them. This book will ensure that all of your meals are delicious and safe to eat. The best part is that the ingredients can be found in most grocery stores, and the step-by-step instructions will make it easy to prepare the meal quickly.

In addition to the recipes, you will also find important transitional information for a gluten- and dairy-free diet in this book, such as how to avoid them in purchased foods and avoid cross contamination. Additionally, you will learn how to avoid gluten and dairy at work and in restaurants. You can also use these recipes to prepare delicious meals with flavour for your family. Prepare to experience improved health and a healthy eating lifestyle.

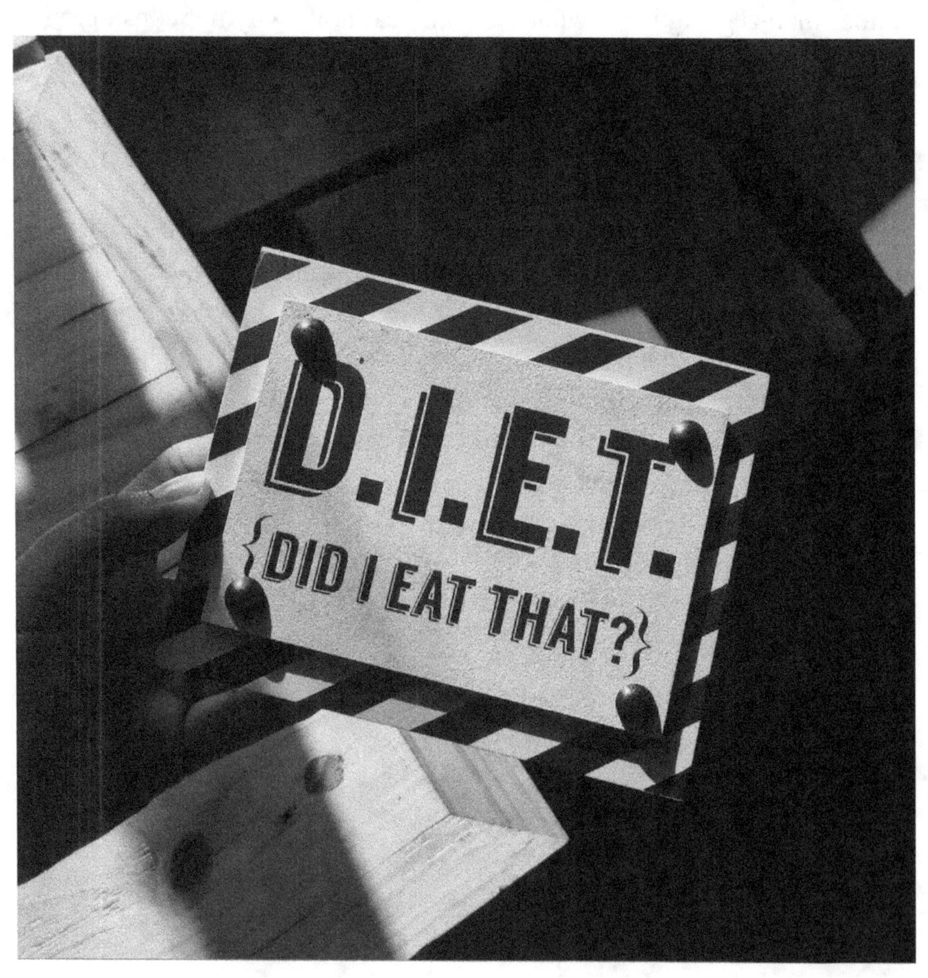

D.I.E.T.
{DID I EAT THAT?}

Chapter One

Food and Supplements

Food is a substance primarily composed of protein, carbohydrates, fat, and other nutrients utilised by an organism's body for energy, vital processes, and growth. Nutrition depends on digestion, which makes it easier for the body to absorb and use food.

Vitamins, minerals, amino acids, fatty acids, and other substances can be taken as food supplements in the form of pills, tablets, capsules, liquid, and so on. Various dosages and combinations of supplements are available. However, our bodies only require a certain amount of each nutrient to function, and higher amounts are not always better. At high portions, a few substances might make unfriendly impacts, and may become destructive. Supplements can only be legally sold with a recommendation for the appropriate daily dose and a warning to not exceed that dose to protect consumers' health.

Food supplements can likewise contain substances that poor people have affirmed as being fundamental for life, yet are showcased as making a valuable natural difference, for example, plant shades or polyphenols. Supplement ingredients like fish or chicken collagen, for instance, can also come from animals. Additionally, these can be purchased separately or in combination with nutrient ingredients. Women are more likely than men to use supplements.

Numerous food supplements are available, but who are they intended for? When are they advantageous, ineffective, or even detrimental? We look at the general advice for taking food supplements in this article.

Who requires dietary supplements?

A well-balanced, nutritious diet cannot be substituted for supplements.
All of the nutrients necessary for good health should typically be found
in a diet rich in fruits, vegetables, whole grains, protein, and healthy
fats. These rules don't mention supplements, but there are some groups
of people or people who might need advice on supplements, even if
they eat a well-balanced diet, like women who are pregnant or on clear
prescriptions.

Gluten free

A gluten-free diet is an eating plan that rejects food varieties containing
gluten. Wheat, barley, rye, and triticale—a cross between wheat and
rye—all contain the protein gluten.

Why eliminate or go gluten-free ?

A gluten-free diet is essential for managing celiac disease and other
gluten-related medical conditions. People who haven't been told they
have a problem with gluten also like to follow a gluten-free diet. The
diet is said to improve health, help people lose weight, and give them
more energy. However, more research is needed. The following medical
allergies form the basis for gluten-free diets:

Celiac disease, gluten causes immune system activity that causes
damage to the small intestine lining in celiac disease. Over time, this
damage prevents food's nutrients from being absorbed. An issue with
the immune system causes celiac disease.

Non-celiac gluten responsiveness, causes a few signs and side effects related with celiac illness — including stomach torment, swelling, the runs, obstruction, "hazy mind," rash or cerebral pain — despite the fact that there is no harm to the tissues of the small digestive tract. Although it is unclear how the process works, studies indicate that the immune system is involved.

Gluten ataxia, an autoimmune condition which impairs muscle control and voluntary muscle movement by affecting particular nerve tissues.

Wheat allergy, like other food allergies, is caused by the immune system thinking that gluten or another protein in wheat is a disease-causing virus or bacteria. An antibody to the protein is produced by the immune system, triggering an immune system response that can cause congestion, difficulty breathing, and other symptoms.

Gluten free ingredients

When following a gluten-free diet, you must carefully consider the foods you consume, their ingredients, and their nutritional value. Naturally gluten-free foods include the following:

Leafy foods, beans, seeds, vegetables and nuts in their regular, natural structures, eggs, lean, non-processed meats, fish and poultry, most low-fat dairy items.

Grains, starches or flours that can be essential for a gluten free diet include:

Amaranth, Arrowroot, Buckwheat, Corn (gluten-free cornmeal, grits, and polenta), Flax, Gluten-Free Flours (rice, soy, corn, potato, and bean flours), Hominy (corn), Millet, Quinoa, Wild Rice, Sorghum, Soy, Tapioca (cassava root), and Teff (grains are not permitted).

Oats, in some instances Although oats are naturally gluten-free, they may be contaminated during production with wheat, barley, or rye. Triticale is a hybrid of wheat and rye. Gluten-free oats and oat products have not been cross-contaminated. Certain individuals with celiac sickness, notwithstanding, can't endure the sans gluten marked oats.

Terms to know about wheat. There are wheat varieties, all of which contain gluten:

Depending on how the wheat is milled or processed, different types of wheat flour are referred to as "Durum," "Einkorn," "Emmer," and "Kamut." Every one of the accompanying flours have gluten:

Gluten-free food labels Gluten-free foods must contain fewer than 20 parts per million of gluten, as required by the U.S. Food and Drug Administration (FDA). Farina is milled wheat that is typically used in hot cereals. Graham flour is a coarse whole-wheat flour. Self-rising flour is also known as phosphate flour. Semolina is the part of milled wheat that is used in pasta and couscous. These labels may be on foods like:

*Food that doesn't naturally contain gluten is a prepared food that doesn't contain any gluten.

*Food that has not been cross-contaminated during production with ingredients that contain gluten.

*Food that has been processed to remove gluten and contains an ingredient that contains gluten.

*Gluten-free labels can be applied to alcoholic beverages containing naturally gluten-free ingredients like grapes or juniper berries.

You need to read the labels on processed foods you buy to find out if they contain gluten. The name of the grain in the content list of the label must be included on the label of any food that contains wheat, barley, rye, or triticale or an ingredient derived from them.

Unless they are marked as gluten-free or made with corn, rice, soy, or another gluten-free grain, the following foods should generally be avoided:

Lager, beer, doorman, heavy (ordinarily contain grain)
Breads
Bulgur wheat
Cakes and pies
Confections
Oats
Fellowship wafers
Treats and saltines
Bread garnishes
French fries
Flavours
Impersonation meat or fish
Malt, malt enhancing and other malt items (grain)
Matzo
Pastas
Sausages and handled lunch meats
Salad dressings
Sauces, including soy sauce (wheat)
Prepared rice blends
Sources of prepared snacks like tortilla chips and potatoes
Self-seasoning poultry
Soups, bouillon or soup blends
Vegetables in sauce

Gluten-free free for self and family

For individuals with celiac illness, specifically, staying away from openness to gluten is significant. If you want to avoid cross-contamination in your own home-cooked meals and avoid gluten-containing meals out, the following advice can help:
* Separately store gluten-free and gluten-containing foods.
*Continue to prepare surfaces and food stockpiling regions clean.
* Thoroughly clean cooking utensils and dishes.
*To prevent cross-contamination, toast bread separately or in the oven.
*If at all possible, read restaurant menus online in advance to ensure that you have options.
*When a restaurant is less crowded and better able to meet your needs, go there early or late.

Living a gluten-free free lifestyle

*Become acclimated to perusing food names when you shop
*Know which liquor to stay away from
*Recall you can in any case appreciate feasts out with loved ones
*Know about cross defilement
*Explore in the kitchen
*Keep in mind, gluten-free feasts can in any case be scrumptious and solid

Chapter Two

Let's begin cooking

Breakfast

Cheesy sausage breakfast casserole

<u>Ingredients</u>

- Nonstick cooking spray
- 2 slices whole-grain or white bread
- ½ pounds of browned and drained bulk sausage
- 3 large eggs
- 1 cup milk
- 1½ teaspoons yellow mustard
- ¼ teaspoons salt
- ⅛ teaspoons ground black pepper
- 2 ounces Cabot Seriously Sharp Cheddar, Cabot 2 Year Cheddar, grated, and about ½ cups
- maple syrup for serving, if desired.

<u>Cooking Directions</u>

- Coat 8-by-10-inch or comparative measured baking dish with nonstick cooking splash.
- Attack little pieces and disperse over the lower part of the dish. Sausage on top.
- In a medium bowl, whisk the eggs until well combined; milk, mustard, salt, and pepper, whisked in. Pour over the sausage and bread. Sprinkle cheddar up and over.

- Heat revealed for 35 to 45 minutes or until set the entire way to focus (blade embedded in focus tells the truth).
- Serve warm showered with maple syrup whenever wanted.

Omelette with vegetables

<u>Ingredients</u>
- eggs
- milk
- butter
- mushrooms
- white onions
- peppers
- cheese
- salt and pepper.

<u>Cooking Directions</u>
- Beat the eggs and dairy
- To begin with, whisk together the eggs and dairy until smooth. Mix the egg whites and yolks completely together.
- Prepare the vegetables In a large sauté pan, melt half of the butter over medium heat. Include the peppers, onion, and mushrooms. Cook until soft, about 5 to 7 minutes. A skillet stuffed with chopped green, red, and mushroom ingredients.
- After the eggs have finished cooking, add the remaining butter to the pan and let it melt. Pour the eggs over the vegetables after lowering the heat to medium or low. Within two to three minutes, allow the eggs to slightly set on the bottom. While tilting the pan to allow the liquidy egg on top to flow underneath, use a spatula to gently push one edge of the egg

upward. Pouring a beaten egg into a skillet containing sautéed mushrooms, onions, and peppers. This should be done all the way around the pan until there is no more liquid. Using a wooden spatula, push the edge of an omelette away from the side of the skillet.

- Add the cheddar
- At the point when the egg is nearly done cooking, sprinkle on the cheddar and permit it to liquefy. An omelette that has been cooked in a skillet The omelette should be folded in half or thirds. Fold the remaining half over itself after removing half of the omelette from the pan halfway onto a plate for ease. Serve immediately with salt and pepper to taste.

Greek yoghurt parfait

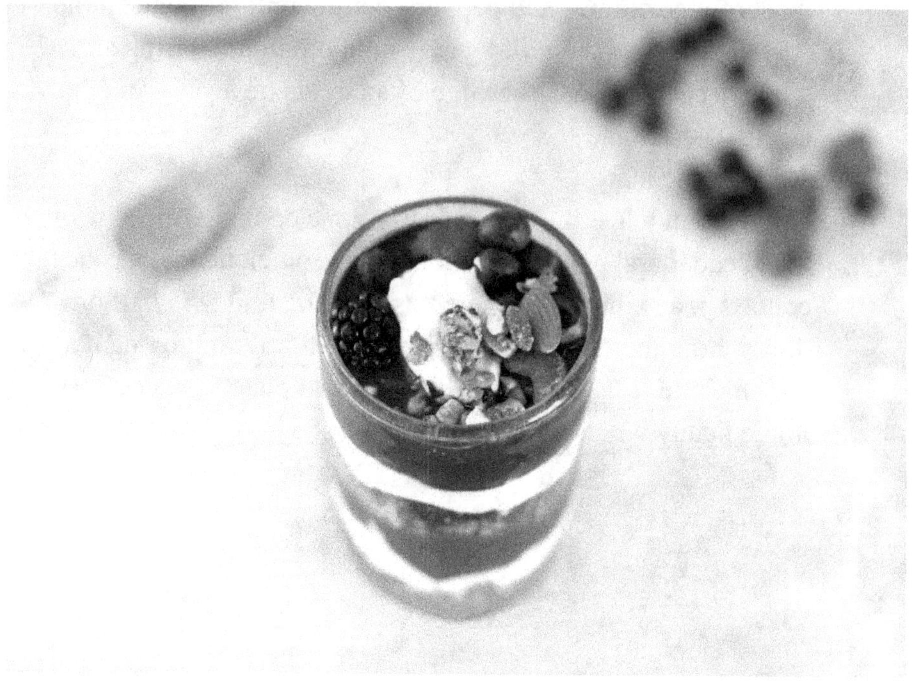

<u>Ingredients</u>

- 10 ounces vanilla greek yoghurt
- 1 cup gluten free granola
- ½ cup pomegranate seeds
- ½ cup blueberries
- 1 tablespoon honey
- ½ tsp chia seeds for embellish

<u>Cooking Directions</u>

Things Required:

Two cups

A spoon (for the yoghurt)

An estimating cup

Estimating spoons

- Take out two cups for the parfaits. Utilising a spoon, scoop two ounces of yoghurt (around two tablespoons) into each cup.
- Using your hands or a clean spoon, evenly distribute the remaining granola into each cup, creating an even layer on top of the granola.
- Take around 50% of the blueberries and pomegranate seeds and do exactly the same thing, separating the two similarly between the cups in an even layer on top of the granola.
- Rehash the layers of yoghurt , granola, and organic product once more. Part the leftover measure of yoghurt (around two ounces) between the cups, putting a spot on top of the organic product.
- Sprinkle a quarter cup of chia seeds and one tablespoon of honey on top of each parfait for decoration. Use a spoon to eat and enjoy!

Avocado toast on gluten-free bread

Toast a slice of gluten-free bread with avocado mash, salt, and pepper, and serve on avocado toast.

<u>Ingredients</u>

2 pieces of gluten-free bread

like Canyon Bakehouse

½ ripe avocado smashed with a fork

2 eggs, fried and cooked to your liking

Coconut oil, for frying

Seasoning salt and pepper
Hot Sauce or tabasco, (optional)

Cooking Directions

- Heat 1 tablespoon of coconut oil in a frying pan over medium heat
- At the point when the oil is hot, add the 2 eggs.
- Add some pepper and salt to taste.
- To ensure that both items are done cooking at the same time, toast the bread.
- Fry the eggs until you like them done
- Placing the toast on a plate
- On each piece of toast, place one egg on top of the mashed avocado.
- On top of everything, sprinkle Everything But The Bagel Seasoning.
- If you want a little more heat, add a little hot sauce. Enjoy!

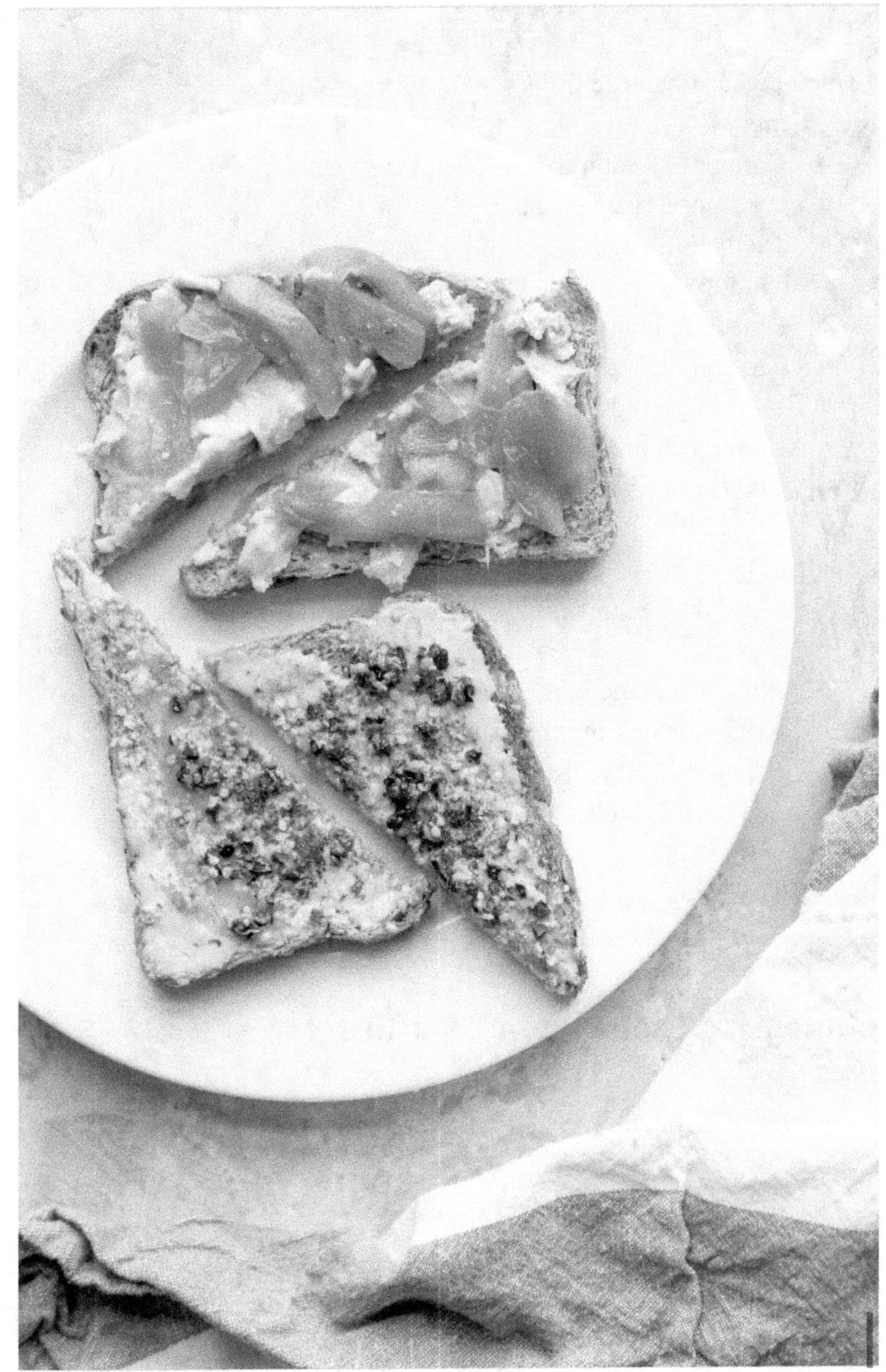

Fruit salad

Combine your favourite fruits

<u>Ingredients</u>

- 1 gram (or 1 tablespoon) of stevia sugar)
- 1 teaspoon rice vinegar
- dried chilli flakes
- cumin
- 1 medium mango
- 1 medium papaya
- 1/4 minced red onion
- 1/2 minced green bell pepper
- 2 tablespoons coriander (finely hacked)

<u>Cooking Directions</u>

- Blend the stevia, vinegar, stew pieces (to taste) and a spot of cumin.
- Add the coriander, papaya, mango, onion, bell pepper, and to avoid crushing the fruit, mix carefully.
- Adjust the salt to taste.
- Serve with chicken or fish as a side dish.

Gluten-free pancakes or waffles

<u>Ingredients</u>

- 2 cups Gluten Free 1-to-1 Baking Flour
- 2 Tbsp Sugar
- 1 tsp Genuine Salt
- 1 ½ tsp Baking Powder

- ½ tsp Baking Pop
- 1 ½-2 cups Water or Milk
- 2 Eggs
- 2 Tbsp Oil or liquefied Margarine (3 Tbsp for waffles)
- 1 tsp Vanilla Concentrate (discretionary)

<u>Cooking Directions</u>
- Preheat a very much oiled skillet over medium-high intensity or preheat a waffle iron as indicated by producer's directions.
- In a medium bowl, join flour, sugar, salt, baking powder and baking pop. Place aside.
- Whisk the eggs, water or milk, oil or melted butter, and vanilla extract (if using) in a large mixing bowl.
- Add the dry ingredients and thoroughly whisk.
- Segment hitter by ¼ cup scoops onto a hot skillet and cook flapjacks 3-5 minutes for each side, until cooked through.
- Cook the waffles according to the manufacturer's instructions. Serve warm.

Breakfast burrito with corn tortilla

<u>Ingredients</u>
- 1 recipe for gluten-free naan (Indian flatbread)
- omitting the baking powder
- 2 large beaten eggs per burrito
- Grated cheddar cheese
- Diced tomatoes (optional)
- Chopped onion (optional)
- Diced bell pepper

- Gluten-free bacon (optional)
- Gluten-free hot sauce or chipotle sauce
- Salt and pepper to taste

Cooking Directions

- Place a sheet of parchment paper or plastic wrap on a flat surface. Plastic melts quickly when placed on a hot skillet, but peeling it off of dough is easier.) Preheat a 10 - 12-inch skillet over medium intensity.
- Sprinkle approximately one to two teaspoons of potato or cornstarch on top of the dough after scooping out 1/4 to 1/3 cup of it onto the parchment or plastic sheet. Pat the mixture out as slight as could really be expected or utilise a starch tidied moving pin.
- Using the plastic or parchment sheet, lift the rolled dough and place it in the heated skillet. Any long pieces of plastic wrap should be tucked behind your fingers.) Fry it for 30 to 60 seconds on each side.
- Rub butter or margarine on the top of the tortilla while it is still in the skillet to keep it soft (this step is optional). You can either stack them between sheets of parchment paper or aluminium foil or place them in a tortilla warmer to keep them warm. Since aluminium foil can get into hot food, I use parchment.)
- When your tortillas are all seared, heat a few oil in a similar skillet and scramble your beaten eggs.
- In a similar skillet, you may likewise saute onions or potentially diced ringer pepper, whenever wanted.
- Add about two scrambled eggs and any desired toppings to each tortilla. Turn the tortilla upside down onto a plate so that it stays closed by folding the ends toward the centre. Serve right away.

- Refrigerate any dough that remains to use the following morning.

Quinoa breakfast bowl

<u>Ingredients</u>
- 1 medium sweet potato that has been peeled and cut into large dices
- Extra-virgin olive oil for drizzling;
- ½ teaspoon of the seasoning of your choice (salt, pepper, etc.).
- 2-2 ½ cups cooked quinoa (⅔- ¾ cup uncooked) adjust amount as desired
- ⅔-1 cup chickpeas
- ½ - ⅔ cups cherry tomatoes, chopped
- 1 avocado (medium), peeled and diced
- 2 scallions, finely chopped, green portion only
- 1 handful spinach leaves (optional)

Protein & Toppings/Garnishes
- Olive oil or dressing of choice
- Juice of ½ lemons
- Sea salt to taste
- Ground black pepper to taste
- 3-4 hard-bubbled eggs, cut or eggs in olive oil
- ⅓ cup chopped parsley

<u>Cooking Directions</u>
- Preheat the oven to 400°F, and line or grease a baking sheet.

- Season the sweet potatoes with your choice of seasonings and toss them with olive oil. Roast until tender and golden, about 20 to 25 minutes.
- In a large bowl, toss the roasted sweet potatoes with cooked quinoa, chickpeas, tomatoes, avocado, scallions, and optional spinach.
- Shower the fixings with olive oil (or a dressing of decision), lemon squeeze, and salt and pepper to taste. Serve in bowls or containers used for meal preparation.
- Sliced hard-boiled or fried eggs should be placed on top of each bowl.
- Add fresh herbs and seasonings of your choice to the bowls.

Tip for Making-Ahead Meals

Make the bowl ingredients (with the exception of the avocado) a day in advance to save time. Divide the ingredients among mason jars or meal prep containers. Just before serving or taking on the go, add the remaining toppings, including the avocado, olive oil, and lemon.

Gluten-free granola and yoghurt

<u>Ingredients</u>

- 1 cup fat-free plain greek yoghurt
- 1/4 cup sliced strawberries
- 2 tablespoons gluten-free granola
- 1 tablespoon honey.

<u>Cooking Directions</u>

- Add 1 cup of yoghurt in a small bowl
- Sliced berries or fruit can be added.

- Drizzle honey or sweetener over the gluten-free granola.

Buckwheat pancakes

<u>Ingredients</u>
- 1 large egg
- 195 g milk 3/4 cup, or non-dairy milk
- 45 g extra-light olive oil 3 tablespoons, or melted butter
- 2 teaspoons of white vinegar or apple cider vinegar
- 1 teaspoon vanilla extract
- 150 g buckwheat flour 1 cup
- 1/2 teaspoon kosher salt
- 1/2 teaspoon baking soda
- 1/4 teaspoon baking powder
- 1 cup blueberries fresh or frozen (optional)
- 3-4 tablespoons butter or non-dairy butter, divided, for the pan

<u>Cooking Directions</u>
- Preheat the oven to 350°F.
- Beat the egg with a fork in a medium bowl or large liquid measuring cup until frothy, about 30 to 60 seconds. To make it vegetarian, skirt this step.
- Utilising a fork, combine the milk, oil or melted butter, vinegar, and vanilla.

- Use a fork to combine the buckwheat flour, salt, baking soda, and baking powder for approximately one minute until just combined. The pancakes won't rise as much if the batter is mixed too much.
- When the skillet is preheated, soften 1 tablespoon of margarine to cover the lower part of the dish. Add more spread on a case by case basis if utilising a bigger frying pan.
- Drop one scoop of batter at a time into the pan with an ice cream scoop or a serving spoon. A 12-inch cast iron skillet will fit 3 flapjacks all at once. When the batter hits the pan, it should sizzle.
- Each pancake should have a heaping tablespoon of blueberries sprinkled on top, and then just enough batter should be added to cover the berries and prevent them from burning when the pancakes are turned over.
- The pancakes should be cooked for about 2 minutes before being flipped over with a spatula. Throughout the process, adjust the heat as necessary.
- Transfer them to a platter that has been warmed under hot water or in a warm oven to keep them warm while the remaining batches are cooked. Cook them for another 1-2 minutes.
- Keep doing this until you've used up all of the buckwheat pancake batter. They are best served warm with butter, warmed maple syrup, and, if desired, fresh fruit.

Breakfast tostadas

<u>Ingredients</u>
- 18 Corn Tortillas (2-3 for each individual)

- Vegetable Oil for broiling
- 12 Entire eggs Around 2 for each individual
- Cooking Shower

<u>Garnishes</u>

Cooked bacon, avocado, cheese, tomatoes, fresh cilantro, green onions, jalapenos, green peppers, salsa, sour cream, hot sauce, lime juice, red onions, pico de gallo, and other options are available to you.

<u>Cooking Directions</u>

- In a large pot, heat about an inch of oil over medium-high heat. When it reaches a sufficient temperature, add the corn tortillas and cook for one to two minutes per tortilla until crisp.
- They must be turned over halfway through. With tongs, remove the tortillas from the pan and place them on paper towels to absorb any excess oil and keep the tortillas crispy.
- If your tortillas do not turn out crispy, you may need to increase the heat. Reduce the heat slightly if they are rapidly burning.

Prepare the toppings next.

Beating ideas: Crispy bacon, avocado, shredded cheese, fresh tomatoes, fresh cilantro, diced green onions, green peppers, salsa (or pico de gallo), red onions, sour cream, hot sauce, and a squeeze of lime juice

- Heat a large frying pan on low to medium heat for the eggs. Apply cooking spray to the pan, then add the eggs and, if desired, a pinch of salt.
- The eggs should be cooked through in one to two minutes. I like scrambled eggs, but there are no rules in this kitchen, so experiment!
- It is now time to put your tostadas together after you have prepared everything! Spread the fixings out "taco bar" style.
- Typically, I begin with a crispy tortilla before adding vegetables, scrambled eggs, and cheese. Enjoy!

Kimchi fried rice

<u>Ingredients</u>

- 2 tablespoons melted coconut or peanut oil
- 1 medium white onion that has been peeled, trimmed, and chopped
- 8 to 16 ounces of kimchi that has been roughly chopped 1½ cups of frozen green peas
- 3 cups of cooked rice that has been chilled
- 1 tablespoon of reduced-sodium tamari
- 1 tablespoon of kimchi brine.

<u>Cooking Directions</u>

- Add the onion and cook until it begins to brown, around 5 minutes. Occasionally stir.
- Add the kimchi and cook until it isn't excessively succulent any longer and is warmed through, around 5 minutes. Cook the green peas until heated through and bright green, about 3 minutes. Place aside.
- To get rid of clumps, use a spoon to break up the rice. Heat the remaining 1 tablespoon of oil on medium-high in a different skillet. Cook the rice in the oil for three minutes or until crisp and heated through.
- Cook for about 2 minutes after adding the kimchi brine and tamari until fragrant and absorbed. Always stir from time to time.
- Combine the vegetables and rice by stirring. Allow the flavours to combine for an additional two minutes.
- Chop dry-roasted peanuts, sesame seeds, thinly sliced scallions, crumbled roasted nori sheet, and/or mild-flavoured fried or baked tofu are some of the options for garnish.

Chilaquiles Verde

<u>Ingredients</u>

- 1 tablespoon olive oil
- ½ large yellow onions diced
- 2 teaspoons minced garlic
- 16 ounces salsa verde
- 1½ ounces corn tortilla chips

<u>Toppings</u>

- 4 large fried eggs
- 1/4 to 1/3 cup crumbled feta cheese or queso fresco
- 1 avocado sliced or diced
- 1-2 radishes sliced
- 14 cup chopped cilantro.

<u>Cooking Directions</u>

- Heat the oil in a large skillet
- Reserve some of the diced onion for later use as a garnish. Cook until tender over medium heat. Stirring in the garlic for about a minute, add it.
- Add the salsa verde, blending, trailed by the stock. Allow to simmer for approximately 5 minutes, or until the salsa thickens, before serving. If you want to fry your eggs in a different pan, this is the best time.
- Season with salt and pepper and eliminate from heat. Stir the tortilla chips in the skillet gently until they are all coated. Cheese, avocado, radishes, onions, cilantro, and chilaquiles are some of the toppings. Serve chilaquiles on plates and top with boiled eggs.

Coconut flour pancakes

<u>Ingredients</u>

For the pancake batter:

Topping (optional):

- 1/4 cup coconut flour
- 1/2 teaspoon baking powder
- a pinch of salt
- 1/3 cup almond milk
- 2 tablespoons of coconut oil, plus additional oil for the skillet's grease.
- 3 beaten eggs
- 2 tablespoons maple syrup
- 1/2 teaspoon pure vanilla extract
- 1 cup fresh fruit
- 4 tablespoons maple syrup

<u>Cooking Directions</u>

- Whisk the Dry Ingredients: In a medium bowl, join coconut flour, baking powder and salt, and blend well.
- Combine the wet components: Almond milk, coconut oil, eggs, maple syrup, and vanilla extract should all be thoroughly combined in a large bowl until the mixture is homogeneous.
- Get ready Hotcake Hitter: Mix well with a hand mixer the dry ingredients into the wet ingredients in a bowl until a consistent pancake batter is achieved.
- Make the pancake batter: Pour 1/4 cup of batter into the middle of a nonstick skillet and heat a little coconut oil over low heat. Batter should cook for about one minute, or until the bottom is golden brown, the top starts to dry out, and bubbles appear. Utilise a non-stick spatula and tenderly flip hotcake to the

opposite side, then let cook for an additional 30 seconds until base is brilliant prior to eliminating. Rehash until everything the hitter is spent.
- Trimming and Serve: Fresh fruit and a generous amount of maple syrup go well with pancakes.

Cowboy breakfast bowl

<u>Ingredients</u>
- 8 slices of bacon
- 2 medium russet potatoes that have been cubed
- 1/4 cup green onions that have been sliced, plus more for garnish
- 3 cloves of minced garlic
- 1 tablespoon paprika
- kosher salt and newly ground dark pepper to taste
- 2 cups cheddar that has been shredded
- 10 eggs that have been scrambled
- 1 avocado that has been sliced
- hot sauce for serving.

<u>Cooking Directions</u>
- Cook the bacon for 8 minutes
- Chop after cooling on a plate lined with paper towels.
- Cook the potatoes in the bacon fat for 10 minutes without stirring, then flip and move around to brown all sides. Add the green onions, and cook for an additional ten minutes until the potatoes are soft.

- Add paprika, garlic, and a generous amount of salt and pepper when the vegetables are tender.
- Add cheddar to potatoes and cover to soften.
- Add scrambled eggs, sliced avocado, cooked bacon, additional scallions, and a drizzle of hot sauce to the cheesy potatoes before assembling.
- Serve and have fun.

Green shakshuka

<u>Ingredients</u>

- 8 tomatillos with their papery husks removed
- 2 cups kale or spinach leaves coarsely chopped
- 1 bunch cilantro coarsely chopped
- 1 jalapeno pepper with its seeds removed and chopped
- 1 tablespoon olive oil
- 1 small white or yellow onion diced
- 2 cloves garlic minced
- 1 15-ounce can of garbanzo beans that have been rinsed and drained
- 1 teaspoon ground cumin
- Kosher or fine sea salt
- Freshly ground black pepper
- 6 large cage-free pastured eggs
- ¼ cup crumbled feta or cotija cheese omit for dairy free

<u>Cooking Directions</u>

- In a large skillet, heat the olive oil to a medium-high temperature. Add the onion and cook until relaxed, around 4 minutes. After being added, cook the garlic for 30 seconds. Cook for about 5 minutes after adding the cumin and garbanzo beans, lightly smashing them with a potato masher or the back of a spoon to keep some texture.

- Add the tomatillo combination to the skillet, bring to a delicate bubble, bring down the intensity and stew, revealed, blending periodically, until the combination thickens and the fluid has vanished, around 25 minutes. Salt and pepper to taste should be added to the mixture.
- Make 6 divots in the combination with the rear of a spoon. Cover the skillet, crack the eggs into the divots, sprinkle with a little salt and pepper, and cook for 6 minutes or until the whites are set.
- Eliminate from heat, sprinkle with cheddar, if utilising, and serve.

Chia pudding

<u>Ingredients</u>

For the pudding

- 4 tablespoons of chia seeds
- 1 cup of your favourite milk (I like: oat milk, cashew milk, coconut milk, and oat milk together
- 1 tablespoon of your choice of liquid sweetener (maple syrup, honey or agave)
- 1 teaspoon unadulterated vanilla concentrate discretionary however suggested

For the Additional items

- Favourite fresh fruit: mango, apricots, berries, and more!

- Nut margarine of decision almond spread, peanut butter, sunflower margarine,

Sprinkle toppings

cut or hacked almonds, toasted coconut chips/drops, cleaved pecans

<u>Cooking Directions</u>
- Whisk together chia seeds and milk in a medium bowl.
- Include the sugar and vanilla concentrate.
- Place in the refrigerator for at least 15 minutes, stirring every 5 minutes to help it thicken.
- Allow to chill in the refrigerator until ready to layer with the Add-On ingredients in a glass.
- In two mason jars (or other containers), layer the toppings of your choice over the thickened Chia Seed Pudding.

Best ever steak and eggs

<u>Ingredients</u>
- 1 or 2 New York Strip steaks that have been trimmed and sliced
- 1 medium onion that has been sliced
- 1 pound of red potatoes that have been peeled and quartered
- 2 tablespoons of canola oil
- 2 tablespoons of butter
- sliced green onions for garnish
- Salt and black pepper.

<u>Cooking Directions</u>
- Season the steak with salt and pepper

- After draining, cook the potatoes in the microwave for six to seven minutes, set them aside.
- Over medium high heat, heat a large cast iron skillet or nonstick skillet. Oil should be added.
- Onions can be fried until the edges turn brown. Include the steak, potatoes, and one tablespoon of butter.
- Cook until potatoes are marginally brown around 5 to 7 minutes then, at that point, season with salt and pepper. Place the remaining butter and 1 tablespoon of oil in a second nonstick skillet and heat over low heat.
- Fry the eggs in twos or one at a time.
- Eggs and green onions should be placed on top of the potato mixture on a platter. If desired, top with steak sauce.

Cinnamon roll baked oats

Ingredients

- 3 cups gluten free oats
- 2 teaspoon baking powder
- 1 ½ tbsp cinnamon
- 2 eggs sub flax eggs for vegetarian
- 1 cup non dairy milk I utilised almond milk
- 1½ tablespoon melted coconut oil
- ¼ cup maple syrup
- ¼ cup brown sugar or coconut sugar
- 1 teaspoon vanilla extract.

Optional icing

- 1-1½ cups powdered sugar
- 1-2 cups water

<u>Cooking Directions</u>

- Line an 8x8-inch baking pan with parchment paper and preheat the oven to 350°F. Combine all of the ingredients in a large bowl until well combined.
- Fill the prepared pan with the mixture, and bake for about 20 minutes. Cool down. Combine the optional icing and drizzle it over the oats. Enjoy!

Chapter Three

Lunch

Quick Guacamole Quinoa Salad for Lunch

<u>Ingredients</u>

- 1 cup uncooked quinoa

- 2 cups water
- 1/2 cup chopped parsley
- 1 medium cucumber
- 1 bell pepper
- 3/4 cup chopped red onion
- 2 avocados peeled and chopped
- 1 cup grape tomatoes

optional other vegetables

- 1/4 cup olive oil
- 1/4 cup lemon juice
- 1 tablespoon red wine vinegar
- 2 cloves garlic pressed or minced
- salt and pepper to taste

<u>Cooking Directions</u>

- Wash the quinoa in a sieve
- In a medium saucepan, add two cups of water.
- Bring to a boil and then reduce to a simmer over medium heat. Uncover and cook for 12 to 15 minutes, or until all of the water has been used up.
- Cover the quinoa for five minutes after taking it off the stove. Allow it to rest so that it expands.
- Join the cucumber, chime pepper, onion, avocado, tomato, and parsley in an enormous blending bowl and put away.
- Using a small whisk, combine the garlic, salt, olive oil, lemon juice, and vinegar in a small bowl.
- Add the cooled quinoa and the dressing to the large bowl of vegetables. Throw to consolidate. season with salt and pepper to taste.
- Serve right away or let it chill for up to three hours.

Rainbow Collard Wraps and Peanut Butter Sauce

<u>Ingredients</u>

- 6-8 large collard green leaves (look for leaves that are larger than your face and have few holes or tears)
- 2 cups chopped romaine
- 2 cups chopped carrots
- 1 cup chopped red bell pepper
- 1 cup chopped yellow mango
- 1 cup chopped avocado
- 1 cup chopped red cabbage
- 1/2 cup chopped english cucumber
- 1/2 cup chopped cilantro
- 1 cup cooked and cooled noodles

<u>Thai peanut sauce</u>

- ¼ cup of water
- ¼ cup of powdered peanut butter
- ¼ C lime juice
- 2 tablespoons rice vinegar
- 2 tablespoons chilli garlic sauce
- 1 tablespoon maple syrup
- 1 tablespoon coconut aminos
- 2 tablespoons chopped peanuts

<u>Cooking Directions</u>

- In a large pot, bring the water to a boil. Each leaf should be immersed in boiling water for ten to fifteen seconds before being transferred to an ice bath right away. Allow to air dry.

- Place a leaf with a horizontal spine on a dry, clean surface. Toppings should be layered in the middle, with lettuce at the end and avocado and mango at the beginning. Roll tightly away from you with the seam side down after folding in the sides. Repeat.
- Make plunging sauce by adding all fixings to a bowl and rushing with a fork. Season as desired.
- Serve the wraps cold with sauce for dipping! can be stored for up to five days in airtight containers for convenient lunches!

Slow-cooker Dinner prep Burrito Bowls

<u>Ingredients</u>

- 4 cups slashed romaine lettuce
- 1 cup cherry or grape tomatoes
- 2 entire chime peppers any tone
- 1 cup cooked earthy coloured rice I utilised Seeds of Progress Earthy coloured Rice and Kale Moment
- 1/2 cluster Pork Carnitas Meat
- 1 cup guacamole

<u>Garnish</u>

- 1 lime
- 4 tbsp green or red onion

<u>Cooking Directions</u>

- Make or Thaw out Pork Carnitas
- Make or Thaw out Pork Carnitas, Prep Vegetables

- Wash and hack romaine lettuce - on the off chance that you didn't buy pre-cut lettuce. Wash, dry, and cut down the middle cherry or grape tomatoes.
- Chop bell peppers after deveining and removing the seeds.

Assemble Meal

Add 1 serving of pork carnitas, 1 cup lettuce, 1/4 cup tomatoes, 1/4 cup chime peppers, and 1/4 cup earthy coloured rice to every feast prep compartment. Include 1/4 cup of guacamole. Add an onion or a lime wedge for decoration.

Spring Roll Bowls

<u>Ingredients</u>

- 2 tablespoons almond butter
- 3 tablespoons coconut aminos
- 1 tablespoon coconut sugar
- 2 tablespoons rice vinegar
- 1 teaspoon garlic powder
- 1 teaspoon ginger powder
- a pinch of salt
- 4 ounces rice vermicelli rice noodles
- 1 tablespoon avocado oil
- 1/2 pound shrimp, peeled and deveined
- 1/2 teaspoon salt
- 1/4 teaspoon black pepper
- 1 halved lime
- 1 tablespoon coconut aminos
- 2 cups green cabbage, shredded
- 1 head romaine lettuce

- ½ cup carrot shredded
- 1 cucumber thin sliced
- 1 tbsp chopped cilantro
- 4-8 mint leaves

<u>Cooking Directions</u>

For the sauce

In a bowl, combine all of the ingredients and thoroughly whisk until a smooth sauce forms. Put away.

For the bowls

- Follow the headings on the bundle to cook the noodles. Set aside after straining and rinsing with cold water.
- Utilising a huge dish, heat the avocado oil over medium intensity. Season with salt and pepper before adding the shrimp. Cook the shrimp for three to four minutes, or until they are pink and cooked through. Add coconut aminos and half of the lime juice to the top. Allow the shrimp to cool slightly before putting it aside and mixing to coat.
- Divide the cooked noodles, shrimp, vegetables, and herbs between two bowls to assemble the bowls. Toss to coat all of the ingredients in the sauce before topping with sauce.
- Present with lime wedges and appreciate!

Cauliflower Fried Rice

<u>Ingredients</u>

1 head of cauliflower should yield 4 cups of rice

1 teaspoon sesame oil

 1/2 yellow onion finely diced

1/2 cup frozen peas or carrots

1/4 teaspoon ground ginger

1 teaspoon red pepper flakes (omit if you don't want it spicy)
2 large cloves of garlic pressed or minced
2 tablespoons soy sauce, tamari, or tamari if gluten-free; 1/2 to 1 tablespoon lime juice
2 tablespoon sliced green onions
2 tablespoon of chopped cilantro

<u>Cooking Directions</u>
- Cut cauliflower into florets
- Wash and dry the florets.
- Place cauliflower into the food processor and heartbeat until it looks like rice.
- Place aside.
- Fried Cauliflower Rice
- Heat oil to a medium temperature.
- Cook the spices, vegetables, and onions for about 5 minutes, or until the vegetables are soft, once the pan is hot.
- In the last 30 seconds, add the garlic.Turn down the heat to medium low.
- Cook the cauliflower "rice" for about 5 minutes or until it reaches the desired texture.
- Mix in soy sauce, lime juice, green onions, and cilantro.Check for seasoning and taste.
- Serve it plain or with chicken, shrimp, or other meats.

Firecracker Chicken with Rice

<u>Ingredients</u>

- Gluten-free nonstick cooking spray
- ½ cup Wholesome Organic Brown Sugar
- ¼ -⅓ cup hot sauce
- 1 tablespoon rice vinegar
- ¼ teaspoon red pepper flakes, if desired
- 6 boneless, skinless chicken thighs
- Kosher or fine sea salt
- black pepper
- ½ cup cornstarch
- 2 large eggs
- lightly beaten
- 3 tablespoons vegetable oil
- 4 cups cooked rice
- 2 sliced green onion

<u>Cooking Directions</u>

- Preheat oven to 350 degrees
- Use cooking spray to spray a baking pan that is 9 by 12 inches
- Sugar, vinegar, red pepper flakes, and hot sauce are all combined in a bowl.
- Make 1-inch-thick cuts in the chicken. Toss the vegetables with salt and pepper to coat. Toss the chicken with the cornstarch in a large bowl to coat. In a large skillet, heat the oil to medium-high heat. In another bowl, place the eggs.
- In a large skillet, heat the oil until it is hot over medium-high heat. Dip a few of the chicken pieces in the egg, shake off the excess, and arrange them evenly in the skillet while working next to the stove. Cook the chicken in batches for 3 to 4 minutes, or until lightly browned. Place in the baking dish you prepared. Add the sauce to the pan after all the chicken has been

cooked, toss to coat, and bake for thirty minutes, stirring halfway through.
- Green onions and rice should be on top.

Oven-roasted Sweet Potatoes with Crispy Chickpeas

<u>Ingredients</u>
- 4 medium sweet potatoes
- 4 tablespoons olive oil
- 1 large garlic clove, crushed
- 1 banana shallot, finely chopped
- 400 grams can chickpeas, drained
- 75 grams baby leaf spinach
- Small bunch dill, finely chopped
- zest and juice 1 lemon

<u>For the tahini yoghurt</u>
- 60 grams Greek yoghurt
- 2 tablespoons tahini
- 20 grams pine nuts, toasted
- 110 grams pomegranate seeds

<u>Cooking Directions</u>
- Fold each potato in a foil and place on the hot coal of a barbecue for 35-45 mins.
- To determine whether they have been cooked, insert a skewer into each one. Alternately, place the potatoes wrapped in foil on a large baking sheet and heat the oven to 200 C/180 C fan/gas 6. The centre should be soft when baked in the oven for 45 to 1

hour. When cooked, put under a hot barbecue for 3 mins until the skin is darkened and fresh.)

- In the meantime, in a large frying pan, heat 1 tablespoonful olive oil over medium heat. Stir the chickpeas into the garlic and shallot mixture after frying for two to three minutes, or until they are soft. After about one minute of gentle heating, add the spinach and allow it to wilt. Include the dill.
- Whisk together the lemon squeeze, zing and remaining olive oil in a little bowl. Mix into the chickpea mixture and season to taste. Use a potato masher to gently mash the chickpeas until they are lightly crushed. Combine as one the yoghurt and tahini in another little bowl, and season to taste with salt.
- Cut the potatoes in half lengthwise. Fill with the bean mixture, top with the pomegranate seeds and pine nuts, and drizzle with tahini yoghurt .

Baked Quinoa Chicken Nuggets

<u>Ingredients</u>

- 1 package chicken breasts, cut into nuggets
- 2 cups cooked quinoa
- 3/4 cup avocado oil (or egg substitute)
- 2 teaspoons garlic powder
- dash salt
- buffalo sauce (optional)
- dipping sauce.

<u>Cooking Directions</u>

- Preheat oven to 400 °F

- Combine cooked quinoa, garlic, salt, and any desired additional spices in a bowl.
- Pour avocado oil (or sub an egg in the event that you can endure) into another bowl.
- Place each piece of chicken on a baking sheet after being dipped in quinoa and avocado oil.
- Prepare for 30-35 minutes, or until firm! Option to broil for one minute at the end for a crispier finish.
- Serve with your favourite sauce for dipping!

Sweet Potato, Bacon, and Broccoli Egg Muffins

<u>Ingredients</u>

- 9 large eggs
- 1 tablespoon ghee or clarified butter, if necessary for the pan
- 2 tablespoons full-fat coconut milk
- 2 tablespoons salsa of choice
- 2 tablespoons nutritional yeast
- salt and black pepper
- 6 slices chopped thick-cut bacon
- 1½ cups shredded sweet potato
- 1 cup finely chopped broccoli florets

<u>Cooking Directions</u>

- Preheat the oven to 400°F. Set out a silicone 12-cup muffin pan or a regular muffin pan that has been greased with ghee. In a bowl, whisk together the eggs, coconut milk, salsa, and nourishing yeast. Add some salt and pepper to taste. Put away.

- The bacon should be cooked in a skillet over medium heat until the fat renders and the bacon is crisp, stirring occasionally. Using a slotted spoon, transfer the bacon to a piece of paper towel. Add the sweet potato and broccoli to the same skillet and cook, stirring, for about 5 minutes until softened.
- Layer the bacon, sweet potato, and broccoli mixture in the cups of the muffin pan. Empty the egg blend similarly into each cup, then, at that point, mix to ensure the fixings are appropriated equitably.
- Bake until set, about 15 to 20 minutes. Cover and keep in the refrigerator for up to three days, or let it cool slightly before serving.

Chickpea and Vegetable Coconut Curry

<u>Ingredients</u>

- 1½tablespoons oil
- 4-5 large garlic cloves chopped
- 1½ inch ginger chopped
- ½ jalapeno chopped, adjust to taste,
- 1 medium red onion chopped
- 14.5 oz can diced tomatoes
- 1 teaspoon The Spice Hunter Coriander Powder
- ½ teaspoon The Spice Hunter Cumin Powder
- ½ teaspoon The Spice Hunter Smoked Paprika
- ½ teaspoon The Spice Hunter Turmeric
- ¾ -1 teaspoon salt to taste,
- 2 cups cauliflower florets
- 1 + 1/4 cup sweet potatoes diced, from 1 medium sweet potato

- 15.5 oz can chickpeas drained
- 1-1½ cups water
- 13.5 oz can coconut milk
- 1 red pepper sliced
- 2 tablespoons chopped cilantro
- ½ lime juice
- ¼ teaspoon garam masala

<u>Cooking Directions</u>

- Heat the oil on a medium heat. Add the chopped ginger, garlic, jalapeño, and onions once the oil is hot. Cook for about 3 minutes until the onion mellows.
- Then add a 14.5 oz container of diced tomatoes and mix. Cover the pot with a top and let the tomatoes cook for 4 to 5 minutes on medium intensity.
- Add 1 teaspoon of Spice Hunter's coriander powder, 1/2 teaspoon of cumin powder, 1/2 teaspoon of smoked paprika, 1/2 teaspoon of turmeric, and salt to taste after the lid has been removed. Cook the spices for one minute with a stir.
- Diced sweet potatoes, a can of chickpeas, and cauliflower florets should be added. Stir until the spices cover the vegetables and chickpeas thoroughly.
- After that, give the can of coconut milk and water a thorough stir. Cover and cook for 10 minutes, mix two or multiple in the middle between.
- Then eliminate cover, add cut ringer peppers. Cook covered for an additional five minutes.
- Eliminate cover, add cleaved cilantro and crush in new lime juice. Put the heat off. Sprinkle garam masala. At this point, the

curry may appear thin, but it will continue to thicken as it cools. Present with earthy coloured rice or jasmine rice!

Fried Eggs and Greens with Sweet Potato Rösiti

<u>Ingredients</u>
- 1 pound sweet potato, stripped and ground
- 1 large shallot, finely minced
- 2 tablespoons earthy coloured rice flour
- 2 tablespoons finely slashed new cilantro
- 1 large egg, softly beaten
- ½ teaspoon fit salt
- ½ teaspoon ground cumin
- Pinch of newly ground dark pepper
- Olive oil, for searing
- 4 large eggs, for searing
- Arugula, to serve

<u>Cooking Directions</u>
- In a huge bowl, blend the potato, shallot, earthy coloured rice flour, cilantro, egg, salt, cumin and pepper.
- Add enough olive oil to coat the bottom of a large skillet heated to medium. Scoop about ¼ cup of the yam into the container, straighten it and broil until firm, around 3 minutes on each side (be mindful so as not to consume it). Transfer the rösti to a plate lined with paper towels with a spatula. Make 12 rosti by repeating the process with the remaining sweet potato mixture.
- In a similar dish, add a shower of olive oil. Add two eggs to the pan and season them with salt and pepper. Fry them for about 5

minutes until the whites are set and the edges are crispy. After removing the eggs from the pan, fry the remaining two eggs. Fried eggs and arugula on top of the rösti are a delicious addition.

Turkey Sausage And Veggie Polenta Bowls

<u>Ingredients</u>

- 1½ lb organic ground turkey sausage
- 6 quartered and chopped carrots,
- 2 red bell peppers,
- 2 zucchini
- 1 head kale, torn or chopped into bite-sized pieces
- 2 teaspoons sea salt
- 2 teaspoons pepper to taste
- Herby Parmesan Polenta

<u>Cooking Directions</u>

- Brown the sausage on all sides in a large stock pot over medium-high heat.
- Add carrots next and let cook for 5-7 minutes prior to adding chime pepper and zucchini.
- Sprinkle it with pepper and sea salt.
- Cook until the kale is wilted by adding it in the last two to three minutes.
- Make the Herby Parmesan Polenta in the meantime.
- Scoop the polenta into bowls and top with the sausage and vegetable mixture when it is ready to serve.
- If desired, top with additional parmesan cheese.

Roasted Tandoori Cauliflower Bowls

Ingredients

- 1 head cauliflower
- 2 teaspoons kashmiri chilli powder
- 1 teaspoon fennel powder
- 1 teaspoon coriander powder
- 1 teaspoon garam masala
- 1 teaspoon onion powder
- 1 teaspoon garlic powder
- ½ teaspoon turmeric
- ½ teaspoon black pepper
- ½ teaspoon lime juice
- 1 teaspoon kasuri methi (fenugreek leaves)
- 2 teaspoons oil
- salt
- 1 teaspoon tandoori masala (optional)
- sprinkle of water (if the pasta is too thick)

Mint-Cilantro Chutney

- 150 g silken tofu
- 1.5 cups mint leaves
- 1 cup cilantro
- 1 tsp garam masala
- 1 tsp minced ginger
- 1-2 green chillies
- salt

<u>Cooking Directions</u>

- Make a thick, smooth paste by combining all of the ingredients.
- Apply it liberally to the cauliflower head. You could also add them to the pasta and quickly toss them after breaking them up.
- Add more oil by spraying or drizzling it on.
- Bake for about 40 to 50 minutes, or until some charring is visible. Spray or drizzle additional oil halfway through baking.
- In the meantime, blend the mint chutney ingredients until smooth. Add some water if the chutney is too thick.
- To serve, garnish the cauliflower with mint chutney and lemon wedges. You might actually decorate with parsley/coriander assuming you'd like.

Chicken And Snap Pea Stir-fry

<u>Ingredients</u>

- 4 cubed, skinless, boneless chicken breasts (about 1.5 pounds).
- ½ pound of fresh snow peas (about 2 cups)
- 4 large cloves of minced garlic
- ¾ cup of coarsely chopped onion
- ⅔ cup of julienne sliced carrots (or celery sliced carrots)
- 3 tablespoons low sodium soy sauce (or smooth)
- 2 teaspoons apple cider vinegar
- 1 teaspoon ground ginger
- 1 teaspoon tapioca flour
- 1½ Tablespoons honey
- 1 Tablespoon extra virgin olive oil
- ¼ cup gluten free chicken broth
- 3 teaspoons of extra virgin olive oil for frying

- Soy sauce, peanut butter, vinegar, ginger, tapioca flour, honey, and olive oil are all combined in a bowl.
- Preheat and oil profound skillet or wok.Add the garlic and chicken; cook the chicken until the outside is no longer pink.
- Add onion, carrots, snow peas and chicken stock; occasionally stir; and cook for three minutes, or until the peas are slightly tender.
- Add sauce combination; stir; and cook for roughly one minute.
- Serve with Shirataki noodles, brown rice, or white rice.

Avocado Chicken Salad

Ingredients

- 1 ripe avocado
- 1 lime juice
- 1 tablespoon greek yoghurt
- 2 diced celery stalks
- ¼ diced red onion
- 1 chilled and chunked chicken breast, sea salt and pepper to taste

Cooking Directions

Mash avocado with greek yoghurt, lime juice, and pinches of sea salt and pepper. Add celery, red onion, and chicken.

Vegan Fiesta Taco Bowl

<u>Ingredients</u>

- ⅓ cup olive oil
- ¼ cup lime juice
- ½ cup chopped fresh cilantro
- 2 tablespoons agave nectar
- 1 seeded jalapeño
- ¼ teaspoon sea salt
- ¼ teaspoon freshly ground black pepper

<u>For the salad</u>

- 2 heads of romaine lettuce, roughly 15 ounces in weight, cut or torn into bite-sized pieces
- 1 cup cooked quinoa
- 1 cup canned dark beans, depleted and flushed
- 1 cup frozen sweet yellow corn, thawed
- 1 cup halved cherry tomatoes
- 1 avocado, mashed
- lime wedges Crispy tortilla strips
- 8 ounces ground seitan
- 2 tablespoons olive oil
- 1 teaspoon chilli powder
- 1 teaspoon smoked paprika
- a pinch of cayenne
- sea salt

<u>For the Lime sour cream</u>

- 1 cup silken tofu
- ¼ cup olive oil
- 2 tablespoons lime juice
- ½ teaspoon sea salt

<u>Cooking Directions</u>

- In a blender or food processor, combine all of the dressing ingredients and blend until smooth. This recipe makes 1 cup of silken tofu, 1/4 cup olive oil, 2 tablespoons lime juice, and 1/2 teaspoon sea salt. Put away.
- In a large skillet, heat the olive oil to a medium temperature. Add the seitan, chilli powder, smoked paprika, and cayenne when it starts to shimmer, and cook until heated through. If the pan appears to be dry, add water one tablespoon at a time. Season with salt.
- To assemble, combine the quinoa, black beans, corn, cherry tomatoes, and sufficient dressing in a large bowl. If you like, garnish each bowl with mashed avocado, smoky seitan, and crispy tortilla strips.
- Blend all of the ingredients for the sour cream in a blender or food processor until smooth. Keep in an airtight container in the refrigerator for up to five days.
- Serve with a lime wedge and lime sour cream in the bowl.

Cold Soba Noodle Salad With Strawberries

<u>Ingredients</u>
Dressing:
- 1 cup rice wine vinegar
- 1 tablespoon sugar
- 1 teaspoon salt
- 2 tablespoons white miso
- 1 hot red chile, finely minced, or more to taste

- 2 tablespoons toasted sesame oil

<u>Salad</u>
- 18 oz package soba noodles, cooked and rinsed
- 4 ounces shishito peppers
- 2 Persian cucumber
- 8 ounces of strawberries
- 1 small red chile, thinly sliced
- 2 scallions, white and green parts, managed and meagerly cut
- ¼ cup fresh mint leaves, roughly chopped
- ¼ cup cilantro leaves

<u>Cooking Directions</u>
Making the dressing
- In a little bowl, join the vinegar, sugar, and salt to disintegrate. Whisk in the miso, chile, and oil to combine. Put away.
- Toss the noodles with the dressing in a serving bowl.
- The shishito peppers should be grilled for three minutes on each side on a hot grill, grill pan, or cast-iron skillet until they are soft and blistered.
- After cooling, slice on the bias, keeping the seeds out.

Put the salad together
- Grilled peppers, cucumbers, strawberries, chilli, scallions, mint, and cilantro should be topped with the dressed noodles; Gently mix to combine.

Chicken Tikka Masala Meatballs

<u>Ingredients</u>

- 1 pound either of ground dark meat chicken or turkey
- 1 large beaten egg
- 2 tablespoons tomato paste
- 1 tablespoon extra virgin olive oil
- ¼ cup finely chopped mint or cilantro
- 1 large shallot minced
- 2 garlic cloves minced
- 2 tablespoons finely minced ginger
- ½ teaspoon ground cumin
- 1 teaspoon sea salt
- ½ gluten-free oat or breadcrumbs

For the sauce

- 2 cups tomato sauce preferably homemade
- 1 tablespoon coconut or olive oil
- 1 large shallot minced
- 1 serrano chilli pepper seeds and ribs removed, minced
- 1½ teaspoon garam masala
- 2 garlic cloves minced
- 1 tablespoon finely minced ginger
- 1 teaspoon ground cumin
- ¼ cup plain full fat Greek yoghurt plus more for serving

<u>Cooking Directions</u>

- Preheat the oven to 400 degrees F. In a large bowl, combine the ground chicken, egg, tomato paste, olive oil, mint, garlic, shallot, ginger, cumin and salt.
- Pulse the oats in a small food processor until they are coarsely ground. Include in the bowl. Mix the chicken with the other

ingredients until it is loosely combined with clean hands. The meat shouldn't be broken up too much. Roll the chicken in your hands until it is smooth and round, then divide it into 2-inch balls using an ice cream scoop. You should have 16 balls, so arrange them on a baking sheet lined with parchment and bake them for 20 to 25 minutes until they are cooked through and starting to brown on the bottom.

Make the sauce in the meantime

- In a large skillet or saucepan, heat the coconut or olive oil. Sauté the shallot, pepper, garlic and ginger over medium intensity until delicate, 3 minutes.
- Incorporate the cumin and garam masala. Continue cooking for two more minutes until the paste is very fragrant. Carefully pour in the tomato sauce.5 minutes, or until the mixture has thickened and the flavours have merged.
- Fold in the Greek yoghurt yoghurt while it is still warm. Check the seasoning and, if you like it hotter, add more salt or a pinch of cayenne.
- Serve the chicken meatballs immediately over brown rice or quinoa with the tikka masala sauce.
- Add chopped mint and additional yoghurt for a garnish.

Walnut seed loaf

<u>Ingredients</u>

- 150 g (1/4 cup) ground walnuts
- 150 g (1/4 cup) gluten-free flour blend (or plain flour if gluten-free)
- 2 heaped teaspoons baking powder

- ¼ teaspoon bicarbonate of soda (to taste)
- ¼ teaspoon salt to taste
- 230 ml unsweetened almond milk
- 1 tablespoon apple cider vinegar

<u>Cooking Directions</u>
- Preheat the stove to 180 degrees Celsius (350 degrees Fahrenheit)
- Place the pecans in a food processor and heartbeat momentarily until you get a fine powder (be mindful so as not to mix excessively, any other way you'll wind up making pecan margarine!)
- In a large bowl, combine the ground walnuts with the gluten-free flour, baking powder, bicarbonate of soda, salt, and milk. Pour the mixture into a loaf pan (I used a one-pound loaf pan) lined with greased baking paper. Sprinkle with mixed seeds to decorate if desired. Bake for 40 to 45 minutes, or until the centre is firm to the touch and a skewer inserted comes out clean. Before storing, cool on a wire rack.

Buffalo-stuffed Sweet Potatoes

<u>Ingredients</u>
- 2 medium chicken breasts that weigh about 1 pound 5 ounces
- 4 large sweet potatoes or 8 small sweet potatoes
- 2 thinly sliced green onions with the white and light green parts separated from the dark green parts

- Creamy Buffalo Sauce
- 3 tablespoons mayonnaise
- 1/2 cup plus
- 1 tablespoon hot sauce like
- 1 tablespoon of Frank's RedHot
- 1/2 teaspoon ranch dressing minced garlic
- 1/2 teaspoon salt

To serve
Add more ranch dressing, celery sticks, or blue cheese crumbles if you're not following a Whole30 or dairy-free diet.

<u>Cooking Directions</u>

- Preheat the oven, Wash sweet potatoes and pierce them all over with a fork. Set up on an oven rack. Salt the chicken breasts thoroughly on both sides. Place in an oven-safe baking dish.
- Remove the chicken from the oven 20 to 25 minutes or when a thermometer inserted into the thickest part of the chicken breast registers 161 degrees Fahrenheit. Bake the sweet potatoes for another 20 to 30 minutes, or until they are soft.
- Chicken should be slightly cooled while sweet potatoes are baking. Shred chicken, either by hand with two forks or with a stand or hand blender. Mix all of the ingredients for the sauce together in a small bowl until smooth. Sprinkle the white and light green parts of sliced green onions over the chicken. Stir well to combine.
- At the point when potatoes are delicate, remove from the stove and cut down the centre cautiously. To slightly open the sweet potato, push the ends in while protecting your hands with a towel or potholder. Fill the cavity with the buffalo chicken

mixture, drizzle more ranch dressing on top, and top with dark green parts of sliced green onions for decoration. Sprinkle with blue cheddar disintegrates whenever wanted (and not on Whole30 or dairy free) and present with celery sticks (discretionary).

Chapter Four

Poultry

Chinese honey chicken

<u>Ingredients</u>
- honey
- gluten-free soy sauce
- apple cider vinegar
- sesame oil
- crushed red pepper flakes
- cornstarch

- brown sugar
- eggs
- olive oil
- Thai chili pepper
- garlic and green onions.

Cooking Directions

- Prepare the sauce. Set aside in a small bowl the honey, gluten-free soy sauce, apple cider vinegar, sesame oil, and red pepper flakes.
- Prepare the chicken's batter station. In a large rimmed plate or shallow bowl, whisk one egg. In a second shallow bowl, combine brown sugar and cornstarch. Dip each chicken piece in the beaten egg. After that, transfer the chicken pieces to the cornstarch mixture, making sure to drain any egg-derived excess liquid before adding the chicken to the cornstarch.
- Let the chicken cook. On the stove, heat olive oil in a large skillet or wok over medium heat. Add the battered chicken, minced garlic, and chilli pepper when the oil is hot.
- Cook until caramelised. The chicken should be golden brown on all sides after 3 to 5 minutes.
- Put the sauce in. Pour the honey sauce over the chicken in the skillet once it has browned on the outside. Cook for 2 to 3 seconds.
- With the sauce, simmer. Cover the skillet and cook the chicken in the honey sauce for 6 to 8 minutes over low heat. If desired, garnish the chicken immediately with diced green onions and sesame seeds by removing the lid.

What to serve it with

White rice, brown rice, quinoa, cauliflower rice, stir-fried vegetables, roasted Asian vegetables, steamed broccoli, green beans, or baby bok choy, lettuce wraps,

Sweet and sour chicken

<u>Ingredients</u>
- ⅔ cup cornstarch
- ¼ teaspoon pepper
- 1½ lbs. boneless, skinless chicken tenders (or chicken breasts) pepper
- ½ tsp. garlic salt
- ¼ cup oil of your choice
- 1 can of (20 oz.)pineapple lumps, depleted

Sauce
- ¾ cup sugar
- ¼ cup ketchup
- ½ cup apple juice vinegar
- 1 tablespoon of gluten-free soy sauce
- I teaspoon Garlic salt

<u>Cooking Directions</u>
- Cut the chicken into chunks by slicing off any excess skin with kitchen shears. I cut mine into chunks about 1.5" to 2" in diameter.
- Place a Ziploc bag the size of a gallon in a bowl and fold the top over to keep it in place. Add pepper, garlic salt, and cornstarch. Shake the bag to combine the contents. You can also do this directly in a bowl without a bag

- Fold the top of the bag over to secure it once more when you put it back in the bowl. Include the chicken pieces. To combine, seal the bag and shake it.
- Add the oil to a large, nonstick skillet. When the oil is hot, add half of the chicken pieces and cook just until brown, however not cooked through, flipping parts of earthy coloured different sides.
- Place the chicken in a 9x13 baking dish after removing it from the pan. For ease of cleanup, I line a glass Pyrex measuring 9 by 13 with aluminium foil.
- Continue with the remaining chicken.
- In the pan, add one can of pineapple chunks, making sure to drain them first. While you make the sauce, place the pan of chicken aside.
- Whisk together the sugar, ketchup, apple cider vinegar, garlic salt, gluten-free soy sauce, and ketchup in a medium bowl. Pour over the pineapple and chicken.
- At 325°, bake for one hour. Remove the chicken from the oven and flip it every 15 minutes with a stir.
- Eliminate from broiler and serve over white or earthy coloured rice.

Bonus

Make a second batch of sauce and add it to a small saucepan if you want more sauce for drizzling. It should be boiling. Over medium heat, whisk constantly, and cook for about 7 minutes until reduced and thickened. Then, at that point, serve close to the completely prepared chicken for those that need extra sauce.

Fried chicken

<u>Ingredients</u>

- Tapioca starch
- Buttermilk
- Red wine vinegar
- Cayenne
- oil

<u>Cooking Directions</u>

- In a large mixing bowl, combine the buttermilk, red wine vinegar, and cayenne pepper. Using a whisk, combine the ingredients until they form a froth. This ought to require around 2 minutes.
- Cover the bowl with the buttermilk mixture and add the raw chicken to the liquid ingredients. Wrap plastic wrap around the bowl.
- In the refrigerator, soak the chicken for 12 hours or overnight in the buttermilk. This makes the meat more delicate and delicious when you fry it.
- Eliminate the chicken and dunk it into the custard starch preparing mix. Coat the chicken by tossing it.
- Heat the oil to 350-375 degrees Fahrenheit in a large 12-inch cast-iron skillet or Dutch oven. Measure the temperature with a digital thermometer. Drop the chicken into the hot oil with care. Be on the lookout for the splattering of hot oil from the pan
- To ensure even cooking on both sides, flip the chicken over with long metal tongs. Depending on whether the chicken is bone-in or boneless, the cooking time will vary.

Honey mustard chicken

<u>Ingredients</u>

- , skinless chicken breasts
- ¼ teaspoon salt
- ¼ teaspoon pepper
- 1 tablespoon olive oil
- a medium onion finely diced
- 2 cloves garlic
- 1 cup chicken stock
- ⅓ cup honey
- ⅓ cup dijon mustard
- ½ teaspoon dried thyme.

<u>Cooking Directions</u>

- Preheat the oven to 175 degrees Celsius. Generously season each chicken breast with salt and pepper on both sides.
- In a cast-iron skillet, heat the olive oil and add the chicken breasts. Sear for three minutes on each side until golden, then transfer the chicken to a plate.
- In a skillet, cook the diced onion and crushed garlic for about 4 minutes, or until the onions begin to soften.
- Whisk the honey and mustard together in a bowl. Before adding the honey-mustard mixture and thyme to the skillet, add the chicken stock and bring it to a boil. Allow all that to stew for 3 to 4 minutes prior to returning the chicken bosoms to the skillet. After covering the chicken with some of the sauce, place the skillet in the oven. Bake for one hour. Sprinkle the chicken with somewhat more thyme prior to serving.

Ultimate Chicken salad

<u>Ingredients</u>

- 1½ to 1¾ pounds cooked chicken breasts
- 3½ to 4 cups chopped or shredded chicken (you can use rotisserie chicken or chicken thighs)
- 1 small or medium apple, peeled, cored, and diced (makes 1 cup)
- 3 celery ribs, chopped
- 1 cup red grapes halved
- ½ cup green onion, chopped,
- ½ cup sliced or slivered almonds,
- 1 tbsp fresh thyme
- 1 tbsp fresh dill
- 1½ cup mayo
- 1 tsp ground mustard
- ¾ tsp salt
- ¾ tsp pepper
- 1 tsp lime juice

<u>Cooking Directions</u>

- Cut the chicken and place in a bowl
- To the chicken's bowl, add diced apple, celery, grapes, and green onion. Combine with a mixer.
- Combine mayonnaise, ground mustard, salt, pepper, and lime juice in a separate bowl. Combine with a mixer.
- Empty mayo combination into the bigger bowl with chicken, and so on. Mix everything together so that the seasoned mayo covers everything.

- Add your cut or fragmented almonds, dill, and thyme. Gently shake. So that they don't get lost in the rest, save these ingredients for the end.)
- Taste. Amount to an extra 1/4 tsp salt and pepper in the event that you like. (I usually do, but it really depends on the mayo I use. Before adding more, taste it.)
- You're prepared to serve! Serve it on top of greens, in a sandwich, or in a salad for a filling and delicious meal!

Crispy gluten-free baked chicken

<u>Ingredients</u>

- Boneless, skinless chicken bosoms - butterfly and pound into cutlets, cut into tenders, or chunks
- Olive oil
- Almond flour or almond feast
- Parmesan cheese, grated
- dried tarragon
- garlic powder
- Italian seasoning
- paprika. You could also try smoked paprika, which also has a great flavour.

<u>Cooking Directions</u>

- Preheat the stove to 425°F. Oil a container with olive oil and put away.
- Start by butterflying your chicken bosoms into chicken cutlets (see underneath to figure out how to make chicken cutlets).

- Using a fork, combine the almond flour, grated parmesan, paprika, Italian seasoning, tarragon, garlic powder, and salt and pepper.
- After you have finished mixing, toss the chicken breast cutlets, nuggets, or tenders with the remaining 1 1/2 tablespoons of olive oil until they are all evenly coated.
- After that, you'll dip each chicken cutlet individually into the almond flour mixture. Use the fork to turn the cutlet over and coat the other side after lightly pressing down. Place the chicken on the greased baking sheet once both sides have been thoroughly coated. Rehash with every cutlet until every one of them is covered with the combination and fit to be prepared.
- Flip the cutlets and bake for an additional 5 to 10 minutes, or until the internal temperature reaches 165 degrees Fahrenheit. Serve the crispy almond flour-baked chicken immediately with lemon wedges and your favourite side dishes.

Slow cooker chicken casserole

<u>Ingredients</u>
- 8 skin-on chicken thighs
- 2 tablespoons runny honey
- salt and pepper to taste
- 1 to 2 teaspoons smoked or unsmoked ground paprika
- 8 rashers of back bacon
- 2 tablespoons olive oil
- a large red onion chopped into sixths
- 2 large yellow or white onions chopped finely
- 1 x cut into sixths

- 200 g washed and trimmed baby carrots
- 1 large parsnip peeled and cut into short lengths
- 200 g button or closed cup mushrooms left whole or cut in half depending on size
- fresh oregano (to taste) finely chopped
- fresh thyme (to taste) finely chopped; and keep some sprigs for the top.
- 2 stock cubes
- 200ml strong vegetable stock

Cooking Directions

- Rub honey, salt, pepper, and paprika into each chicken skin.
- Heat the oil to medium-high in the dish for the sluggish cooker in the event that it very well may be utilised on the hob (or in a huge skillet in the event that it can't) and delicately seal and brown the beyond the carefully prepared chicken (around 5 to 8 minutes), turning habitually. Put away.
- Saute the bacon and onions in the same pan for about 5 minutes, or until they start to soften.
- Sauté the mushrooms, carrots, and parsnip for an additional 5 minutes to brown slightly.
- Toss in the chopped herbs and mix well.At this point, transfer the vegetable-bacon mixture to the slow cooker if you are using a separate pan. Utilise some stock to wash round the container to get the juices).
- Place the chicken, skin-side down, directly on top of the vegetables and cover with the stock.
- Cover the surface with some fresh thyme sprigs and close the container.

- Slow cook as indicated by the producer's guidelines for around 3 hours (high) or 6 hours (low).

Gluten Free Custom made Chicken Noodle Soup

<u>Ingredients</u>

- 1 Tablespoon additional virgin olive oil
- 1 Tablespoon spread
- 1 huge or 2 medium carrots, stripped then cut
- 1 stem celery, cut
- 1 shallot or 1/2 little onion, cleaved
- salt and pepper
- 2 cloves garlic, minced
- 64 oz chicken stock, in addition to something else for warming
- 1 chicken bosom, cleaved into scaled down pieces
- 8 oz gluten free spaghetti, broken into pieces (or any easy route pasta)

<u>Cooking Directions</u>

- Heat olive oil and spread in a huge soup pot or Dutch Stove over medium intensity. Add carrots, celery, and shallot, season with salt and pepper, then saute until delicate, 10 minutes. Add the garlic, and cook briefly. Add chicken stock then heat to the point of boiling.
- Add the pasta and salt and pepper-seasoned chicken to boiling chicken broth. Turn heat down to medium then stew, mixing sometimes, until pasta is cooked through. Taste, make any necessary adjustments to the salt and pepper, and then serve.

Korean hot chicken

<u>Ingredients</u>

- 600 g boneless, skinless chicken thigh meat, sliced into medium pieces
- 1/4 teaspoon salt
- 2 teaspoons coconut oil

For the hot sauce

- 1/2 little red onion, generally diced
- 2cm long new ginger root, stripped and generally diced
- 2 cloves garlic, stripped and generally diced
- 1 tablespoon fish sauce
- 3 tablespoons tamari sauce (or coconut aminos)
- 1 teaspoon sesame oil
- 2 tablespoons honey
- 1 tablespoon mirin or rice wine
- 3 teaspoons Korean red powder
- 1 tablespoon tomato glue
- 4 tablespoons water
- 1 tablespoon lemon juice

Garnish

- 2 tablespoons sesame seeds
- Hacked spring onions/scallions

<u>Cooking Directions</u>

- Season the chicken with a touch of ocean salt and put away.
- Blend or process the sauce ingredients in a food processor. Mix together until genuinely smooth, then, at that point, scratch into

a little pan. Grate the onion, ginger, and garlic and thoroughly combine them with the remaining ingredients if you don't have a blender.

- Sesame seeds should be added to a clean frying pan. Heat in a medium-sized pan. Toast the seeds for a few seconds, stirring frequently, until they begin to slightly brown. Place in a bowl.
- Heat a dab of coconut oil in a huge skillet. Cook the chicken pieces for 5 minutes on each side over medium-high heat.
- Set the sauce-filled pot on medium heat while you wait. Stir frequently for approximately two minutes after bringing to a simmer. This will cook some of the ingredients, like ginger, onion, and garlic, which will make their flavours more subtle and thicken the sauce.
- Stir the sauce into the chicken after it has been cooked on each side. Stirring a few times, cook the mixture for two to three minutes. The sauce will caramelise and get considerably more tacky. Lastly, toss in some of the sesame seeds and mix well. The remaining sesame seeds and green onion should be added on top.
- Greens and cauliflower or white rice, if desired, are optional.

Basil-lemon chicken marinade

<u>Ingredients</u>

- Dried basil can be filled in for fresh basil.
- Fresh lemon juice
- Olive oil can be substituted for a neutral vegetable oil
- Chicken:

<u>Cooking Directions</u>

- Put the lemon's zest in a bowl. Incorporate the juice of one lemon. Shred basil leaves with your hands to include 4. Season with salt and pepper. Use olive oil and mix
- Place one of the plastic freezer bags inside the other. In the inner bag, place the chicken.
- Pour over the marinade for the lemon chicken. After making a knot in the bags, massage the chicken through them to distribute the marinade evenly. Refrigerate for at least one hour, turning once halfway through 11, in a bowl.
- Remove the chicken from the marinade and bring it out. Cook the chicken, permit to rest for a couple of moments, and serve

Chapter Five

Beef and Pork

Beef and pork meatballs

<u>Ingredients</u>
Meatballs:

- 1 kilogram mince
- 400 grams gluten-free sausage meat (squeeze it out of six sausages if that's easier)
- 2 tablespoons oil
- 3 slices of gluten-free bread (100 grams)

- 1 tablespoon fresh flat parsley (chopped)
- 1 tablespoon fresh oregano (chopped)
- 1 onion (finely chopped)
- Seasoning to taste

Tomato sauce

- 2 tablespoons oil
- 4 crushed garlic cloves
- 1 tablespoon chopped basil
- 4 cans chopped tomatoes
- 1 tablespoon sugar
- 1 tablespoon of fresh basil
- Seasoning to taste

Cooking Directions

- Set the oven temperature to 220°C. In a large mixing bowl, combine the remaining ingredients for the meatballs with one tablespoon of the oil. Use your fingers to combine. The meatballs will be more tender if you squeeze the mixture well. Form 25 to 30 meatballs and distribute them on two baking trays. To cover the meatballs and prevent them from sticking, drizzle on the remaining oil and gently shake the trays. The meatballs should be cooked through and browned in the oven for 35 to 40 minutes

Tomato sauce

- Heat the oil in a saucepan over medium heat while the meatballs cook. Garlic should be stir-fried for about two minutes. Add different fixings and season to taste. Mix thoroughly. After bringing to a boil, simmer for 15 to 20 minutes to allow the sauce to slightly thicken. Mix every so often

Cabbage with apple and pork broil

<u>Ingredients</u>

- ½ medium head of cabbage, cored and hacked
- 3 cored and diced apples (with the skin on)
- ½ little onion, slashed
- 2 tbsp juice vinegar
- ¼ cup sugar
- ½ tsp salt
- run nutmeg
- Bay leaf
- 1½ lb boneless pork cook, cut back of apparent excess

<u>Cooking Directions</u>

- In a 4.5-qt slow cooker, join all fixings with the exception of pork dish and mix. If you think there isn't enough room for your roast, mash it down a little (the cabbage will cook down a lot while it looks full at first). On top, place the unseasoned roast. Roast should be cooked for at least 160 degrees in the centre when cooked on low for about 8 hours.

Taco filling

<u>Ingredients</u>

- 1 tablespoon extra-light olive oil
- 1 medium onion
- 2 teaspoons chopped garlic
- 1 pound of extra-lean ground beef
- 2 cups cooked pinto beans
- 1 cup tomato sauce, and one can (6 ounces). tomato glue

- 1 cup water
- 1 tbsp taco preparing

<u>Cooking Directions</u>
- Fry the onion and garlic in the olive oil.
- Cook the ground beef until no longer pink by adding it.
- Cook on low until the sauce thickens and the flavours combine and is heated through.
- Use it in tacos, salad, taco pie, and taco potatoes…

Slow-roasted pork loin (crockpot)

<u>Ingredients</u>
- 1 1.5-pound pork loin
- 3 cups chicken stock
- 1 cup white wine
- 1 large onion
- 4 cloves of garlic
- salt and pepper to taste
- 2 tablespoons cornstarch

<u>Cooking Directions</u>
- Place sliced onion in a crockpot.
- Place chopped or crushed garlic in the slow cooker.
- Crockpot should have wine and chicken stock.
- Salt and pepper the loin of pork. Add to the slow cooker.
- Follow the crockpot's instructions to set it up. Let sluggishly cook for somewhere around 6 hours.

- Remove meat from the slow cooker. In a saucepan, add the liquids and bring to a boil.
- Combine ½-3/4 cup of warm water and cornstarch. Add to the boiling liquid. Stir until it becomes thick.

Serving Ideas: I pair the pork loin with rice or mashed potatoes. You can also cook the meat all day in the crockpot with vegetables like mushrooms, carrots, or other vegetables.

Chapter Six

Seafood

Easy Cajun Baked Salmon

<u>Ingredients</u>
- 4 Atlantic, 5 oz. salmon fillets each)
- 1½ teaspoon spread
- 1 tsp.paprika
- ¼ teaspoon dried thyme leaves
- ¼ tsp. dried oregano.
- ¼ tsp. garlic powder
- ¼ tsp. dried parsley
- ⅛ teaspoon onion powder
- ⅛ teaspoon cumin cayenne pepper

- ¼ teaspoon (or to taste)
- ¼ teaspoon packed brown sugar salt
- ¼ teaspoon black pepper

<u>Cooking Directions</u>
- Preheat the oven to 400°F.
- Line a baking sheet with parchment paper.
- With paper towels, gently pat the salmon fillets dry. Put the skin side down on the baking sheet.
- Place the spread in a little microwave-safe bowl. Microwave for about 20 seconds on high until melted.
- Place the paprika, thyme leaves, oregano, parsley, garlic powder, onion powder, cumin, cayenne pepper, sugar, salt, and dark pepper in the bowl with the margarine. Mix with a fork until a thick glue structures.
- Spread about a teaspoon of the spice mixture evenly over the top of each salmon fillet with a clean spoon.
- Split a lemon in half. Apply the juice from one half to the fillets in an even layer. The remaining half can be served.
- Heat the salmon on the centre rack of the broiler until it pieces effectively with a fork, 12-15 minutes.
- Verify that the salmon is done. Alternately, remove from the oven and increase time.
- Crush the saved lemon over the fillets and serve right away. For up to two days, store leftovers in an airtight container in the refrigerator.

Baked garlic butter shrimp scampi

<u>Ingredients</u>

- nonstick cooking shower
- 1 1/2 lb. raw shrimp peeled
- 3/4 teaspoon salt
- black pepper to taste
- 6 Tbsp. melted unsalted butter,
- 4 minced garlic cloves,
- 2 tablespoons grated Parmesan cheese for shrimp
- 3 tablespoons ground Parmesan cheddar (for serving)
- 1 Tbsp. fresh parsley (minced)

<u>Cooking Directions</u>

- Preheat the oven to 375°F. Splash a 9x13-inch baking dish with a nonstick cooking shower.
- Organise the shrimp in an even layer in the baking dish. Add salt and black pepper to taste. Garlic and grated Parmesan cheese are added to the melted butter and shrimp. Use a rubber spatula to toss to coat.
- Bake the shrimp for 8 to 10 minutes on the middle rack of the oven until just opaque. Do not bake for too long.
- Verify that the shrimp is done. Eliminate from broiler or add time depending on the situation.
- Sprinkle the shrimp with the minced parsley and Parmesan cheese. Serve right away.

Grilled bacon wrapped tilapia

<u>Ingredients</u>

- Tilapia fillets
- 8 long, thick slices of raw bacon
- Olive oil
- Salt and pepper to taste
- Garnish with parsley

<u>Cooking Directions</u>
- Preheat the grill to 400 degrees Fahrenheit
- Spray a grilling basket with cooking spray
- Prepare a dish for the tilapia. Cover with salt and pepper.
- Apply a thin coating of olive oil to the fish.
- Take two crude bits of bacon and fold it over the tilapia.
- Do this with each of the bits of tilapia.
- Put into the barbecuing confine.
- To prevent the fish from dripping all over the kitchen, I kept a plate underneath the basket.
- Place the fish in a grill basket on the grill.
- On high heat, cook one side for 5 minutes before flipping the basket to cook the other side.
- Cook until the fish is flaky and white. It's okay if bacon needs a few extra minutes.
- Serves warm and sprinkled with parsley.

Easy rainbow chard curried tuna salad

<u>Ingredients</u>
- 1 cup chopped Swiss chard stems
- 2 cans of tuna fish packed in water, drained
- 3 tablespoons scallions or onion

- 3 tablespoons sunflower seeds
- 1 cup raisins or golden raisins
- 1 cup shredded carrots
- 1 cup regular or vegan mayonnaise
- 2 teaspoons curry powder
- salt and pepper to taste.

<u>Cooking Directions</u>

Combine all of the ingredients in a large bowl thoroughly. Sandwiches, Swiss chard leaves, or lettuce can all be served chilled.

Air fryer cod

<u>Ingredients</u>

- 1½ pounds of cod
- ¼ cup regular or gluten-free flour
- 3 tablespoons plantain flour or more flour
- 2 teaspoons cajun seasoning or old bay
- 1 teaspoon smoked paprika
- ½ teaspoons garlic powder
- ⅛ teaspoons salt
- 1 teaspoon light oil for spraying
- pepper to taste

<u>Cooking Directions</u>

- Spray oil on the basket of the air fryer and heat it to 360 degrees F.
- Wipe the cod dry with a paper towel after taking it out of the package.

- After dipping each piece of fish in the flour-and-spice mixture, turn it over and press down on it to coat it all.
- Place the fish in the crate of the air fryer. Shower with oil. Ensure there is space around each piece of fish so air can circle around the fish.
- Cook each side for 6 to 8 minutes at 360 degrees F. Keep in mind that the amount of time it takes to cook your cod depends on how thick it is! Cook for five minutes on each side for thinner fillets.
- Serve with lemon.

Crispy gluten free fish sticks

<u>Ingredients</u>

- 1 egg
- 2 tablespoons milk
- 1 tablespoon light oil
- salt and pepper to taste
- 12 ounces cod fillets
- 1 cup pork rinds
- salt and pepper to taste

<u>Cooking Directions</u>

- Slice the cod into sticks with a sharp knife.
- In a bowl, combine the egg and milk. Turn the fish around in the mixture after adding it so that all sides are coated.

- Put the fish into the pork skin panko. Ensure it is covered all over.
- Lightly coat the warm air fryer basket with oil. They won't be able to stick as a result of this. Olive oil is not permitted. Place the fish sticks in the air fryer bin, then splash the highest points of the fish sticks with the oil.
- Cook the fish sticks for 10 to 12 minutes at 375 degrees F. You may need to cook your fish sticks for an additional couple of minutes if they are thick.

Smoked Salmon Risotto

<u>Ingredients</u>

- 1½ cups arborio rice
- 2 tablespoons olive oil
- 1 minced clove of garlic
- ½ cup smoked salmon
- ¼ cup chopped scallions
- ½ cup white wine
- 14 fluid ounces low sodium chicken broth
- salt to taste
- 8 sliced fresh shiitake mushrooms
- ¼ cup heavy cream
- ¼ cup grated parmesan cheese.

<u>Cooking Directions</u>

- In a cast-iron skillet, heat olive oil to a medium temperature. Throw in the rice to cover it in the oil. Quickly add the wine and cook until it is completely absorbed.
- Saute mushrooms and scallions for three minutes. Reduce the temperature to a simmer.
- Add ½ cups of chicken broth, and let it simmer. Continue adding chicken broth and simmering it until the rice becomes tender. After three times adding liquid, add smoked salmon.
- Add the cream and parmesan cheese to the rice when it is tender. Blend well. Reduce heat until the rice is creamy. Add salt to taste.

Tuna avocado salad

<u>Ingredients</u>

- 1 can Bella Portofino Fish
- ¼ cup bok choy hacked
- ¼ cup cherry tomatoes hacked
- 3 tablespoons mayonnaise
- ¼ cup hacked carrot
- salt and pepper to taste
- 1 huge avocado

<u>Cooking Directions</u>

- Combine all of the ingredients in a bowl and thoroughly blend.
- Remove the pit from a large avocado by cutting it in half lengthwise.

- Add a scoop of the fish salad into the avocado. Slices of jalapeno may be added as a garnish.

Grilled Alaska halibut with fresh pesto

<u>Ingredients</u>
- Alaska halibut steaks
- 1 teaspoon olive oil (for brushing on fish)
- 1½ cups fresh basil leaves
- 2 cloves garlic
- 3 tablespoons olive oil
- 3 tablespoons toasted pine nuts
- 3 tablespoons parmesan cheese
- ⅛ teaspoon salt
- dash of black pepper

<u>Cooking Directions</u>
- Preheat the grill to 375 degrees Fahrenheit.
- Spread the thawed halibut steaks Use olive oil to brush.
- In a Cuisinart, combine the parmesan cheese, three tablespoons of olive oil, garlic, pine nuts, and basil. Mix well.
- Brush the pesto on the two sides of the fish. Return the fish to the foil.
- With the foil, place the fish on the grill. After the lid is removed, cook for ten minutes.
- Serve quickly.

New England style fish chowder

<u>Ingredients</u>

- 6 cups Clover Lactose Free Entire Milk
- 3 cod fillets
- 2 cloves garlic minced
- 1 cup onion diced
- 2 cups potatoes diced
- 5 cuts bacon cooked, slashed
- 1 teaspoon salt
- 1 teaspoon paprika
- 1 tablespoon new savvy
- 1 tablespoon new thyme
- 1 tablespoon olive oil
- 2 tablespoons cornstarch

<u>Cooking Directions</u>

- In a skillet, add oil and onion. Sauté the onions until they begin to become translucent.
- Add potatoes and cooked bacon. Blend well.
- Cook for ten minutes after adding the cornstarch and seasonings.
- Next, add the cod fillets and milk. The cod fillets can be added whole because they will break up when cooked. If your fish hasn't been defrosted, you can also put it in the freezer.)
- Cover, bring to a boil over medium heat, and simmer for ten minutes.
- Reduce the heat to a simmer and cook for another 20 minutes until the dish is finished.

Honey garlic shrimp marinade

<u>Ingredients</u>

1 pound of shrimp

⅓ cups of honey

¼ cups of coconut aminos

1 tablespoon crushed garlic

1 tablespoon of olive oil.

For the honey garlic shrimp bowls

1 chopped avocado

½ cups of red onion

½ chopped mangoes

1 cup cherry tomatoes

<u>Cooking Directions</u>

- Whisk the marinade together, then cover the shrimp with the liquid and refrigerate for 30 minutes.
- Remove the shrimp from the marinade and keep it aside.
- Eliminate shrimp from the marinade and cook for a couple of moments each side in a lubed skillet.
- Cook the marinade just for 5-7 minutes in a skillet, then add the cooked shrimp and mix well to cover them.

Make honey garlic shrimp bowl

- Follow the instructions above to cook the shrimp.
- Serve shrimp in a bowl with the simple salsa made with mango, cherry tomatoes, red onions, and any other vegetables you like.

Chapter Seven

Sides, Sauces and Dressings

Gluten is a protein that can be found in the majority of foods that are made with grains. It adds elasticity to foods and acts as a binder to keep them together (imagine a soft, pullable sourdough loaf).

Luckily, without gluten options for wheat-filled top choices like bread and pasta are genuinely easy to find in your nearby supermarket. Look no further for ideas for your next dinner party or family meal that are gluten-free! Everyone will enjoy these gluten-free side dishes.

Grilled zucchini with chile mint vinaigrette

<u>Ingredients</u>

- ¼ cup extra-virgin olive oil, in addition to something else for brushing
- 1 fresno chile or ½ jalapeño, meagerly cut
- 1 little garlic clove, meagerly cut
- 1 tablespoon red wine vinegar

- 1 tablespoon new lemon juice (from ½ lemon)
- 1 tablespoon finely cleaved new mint
- 1 teaspoon ground lemon strip (from 1 lemon)
- ½ teaspoon Jewel Precious stone fit salt
- ¼ teaspoon newly ground pepper
- 4 zucchini or yellow squash
- Flaky ocean salt
- ½ cup cherry tomatoes, cut down the middle
- New mint leaves (decorate)

Cooking Directions

- Prepare a medium-high-heat barbecue grill. Whisk together oil, onion, chilli, garlic, red wine vinegar, lemon juice, mint, lemon strip, salt, and pepper in a little bowl. Put vinaigrette away.
- Slice the zucchini in half lengthwise to a thickness of 14 inch, leaving some of the stem on for decoration. Apply oil and sea salt to the brush. The zucchini should be grilled for 5 to 7 minutes, turning once, until it is lightly charred. On a platter, arrange the zucchini; shower with half of the vinaigrette, adding more whenever wanted. Sprinkle it with mint leaves and tomatoes.

Gluten free cauliflower tabbouleh

Ingredients

- 1 head cauliflower or 1 pack frozen cauliflower rice
- 3 medium cucumbers, diced
- 2 celery stems, diced
- 2 stalks green onion, cut utilising both the white and green parts

- ½ cup dried cranberries
- ½ cup parsley, hacked
- ½ cup cilantro, hacked
- 4 tablespoons cut almond
- 2 tablespoons sesame seeds
- lemon and mustard seed vinaigrette (beneath)

Lemon and Mustard Seed Vinaigrette

- ¼ cup olive oil
- zing from ½ lemon
- 3 tablespoons lemon juice
- 1 tablespoon apple juice vinegar
- 1 teaspoon mustard
- 1 teaspoon honey
- salt and pepper

Cooking Directions

- Cauliflower that is fresh: Cauliflower should be boiled for exactly 2 minutes in salted water. Cauliflower should be strained until it is dry, then pulse it in a food processor until it resembles a small bulgur grain.
- Prepare the frozen cauliflower rice according to the instructions on the package. Defrosting the cauliflower in a large nonstick pan until it is cooked through is typically all that is required for this.
- In a large bowl, combine all of the ingredients, excluding the dressing and sesame seeds. Toss to blend.
- Toss to evenly coat with dressing before serving. Then, for a beautiful presentation, sprinkle it with sesame seeds.

Spring crudités with green goddess dressing

<u>Ingredients</u>

- 1 cup whole milk Greek yoghurt
- 1 cup parsley
- 1 cup mixed soft leafy herbs (dill, mint, tarragon, or cilantro)
- 2 tablespoons chopped chives
- 2 tablespoons lemon juice, in addition to ½ teaspoon zing
- 1 tablespoon extra-virgin olive oil
- 2 teaspoons capers
- 1 garlic clove,
- ¼ teaspoon sea salt,
- freshly ground black pepper. cut crude or potentially broiled vegetables

<u>Cooking Directions</u>

- To make the Dressing for the Green Goddess: The yoghurt , parsley, mixed herbs, chives, olive oil, lemon juice, zest, capers, garlic, salt, and pepper should all be combined in a food processor. Pulse until thoroughly mixed. Season as desired.
- Place spring vegetables on a platter and drizzle with Green Goddess Dressing for the crudités. Eat!
- Green Goddess Dressing can be kept for up to five days in the refrigerator in an airtight container.

Sweet and sour cider glazed Brussels sprouts with dates and pecans

<u>Ingredients</u>

- 1 pound of shredded Brussels sprouts, cut into thin slices with a sharp knife
- ¼ cup pitted dates, chopped
- extra virgin olive oil
- kosher salt
- freshly ground black pepper
- 1 cup apple cider
- 2 tablespoons apple cider vinegar
- 1 to 2 tablespoons maple syrup
- ¼ cup toasted pecans; optional
- for using red pepper flakes

<u>Cooking Directions</u>

- Add just enough olive oil to coat the bottom of a large cast iron skillet over high heat. Spread the brussels sprouts out so that as much of their surface area as possible comes into contact with the hot pan before adding them in an even layer.
- Burn without moving, until they start to roast (around 4 minutes.) Give the dates, cider, vinegar, maple syrup, a good pinch of salt and pepper, and the pan a good stir. For another two or three minutes, continue searing the Brussels sprouts until more of them have developed a char. If the sauce reduces too much, add a splash more cider so that it covers the brussels sprouts.
- Place in a serving dish, sprinkle with toasted pecans, season with additional salt and pepper if necessary, and serve. Eat!

Spring herb strawberry and arugula salad with goat cheese and spring herbs

<u>Ingredients</u>

For the dressing:

- 8 cups baby arugula
- 12 stemmed and quartered strawberries
- 1 large peach or nectarine sliced
- ¼ cup chopped candied pecans or walnuts
- ½ cup crumbled goat cheese
- ½ cup chopped mint or basil.
- zing and juice of one lemon
- 1 teaspoon honey
- 1 teaspoon dijon mustard
- 1 teaspoon white wine vinegar
- ¼ cup extra-virgin olive oil
- salt and pepper

<u>Cooking Directions</u>

- Blend all of the ingredients together in a blender or shake them up in a jar with a lid to make the dressing.
- Toss the arugula with a few tablespoons of the vinaigrette in a large bowl. Layer with goat cheese, nuts, strawberries, peach slices, and herbs on a serving platter.
- Sprinkle with salt and pepper, drizzle another tablespoon of dressing over the top, and serve!

Mango and Feta Salad

<u>Ingredients</u>

- 1 cubed avocado
- 6 ounces of cubed feta
- handful of mint
- handful of chives
- handful of basil
- ¼ cup of chopped pistachios
- juice of ½ lemon
- 2 tablespoons good olive oil
- flakey salt to taste
- fresh ground black pepper to taste

<u>Cooking Directions</u>

- Toss the ingredients together in a mixing bowl to ensure that the olive oil and lemon juice cover everything.
- change lemon squeeze or salt/pepper depending on the situation. enjoy!

Crispy potatoes with salt and vinegar

<u>Ingredients</u>

- extra-virgin olive oil
- 1/4 cup apple cider vinegar, plus more for drizzling,
- 1-2 pounds of halved baby potatoes
- Kosher salt and freshly ground black pepper
- chopped chives for garnish.

<u>Cooking Directions</u>

- In an enormous cast iron skillet, add sufficient olive oil to cover the base by around 1/4 inch. Sprinkle an even layer of salt and a few grinds of black pepper on the pan's bottom and heat on medium until it shimmers. Place the potatoes, cut side down, in the pan and cook for ten minutes without stirring.
- At the point when the cut side of the potatoes has cooked, go intensity to low, add 1/4 cup vinegar to the container, and cover.
- Cover and cook for 15 minutes. When they are tender inside, you will know they are finished. Transfer to a dish for serving. Add a pinch of flaky salt, chives, and a few more tablespoons of vinegar to the drizzle if you like. Enjoy!

White bean and radicchio salad

<u>Ingredients</u>

- 1 cup of dried cannellini beans that have been soaked overnight in water
- 1 shallot that has been finely diced
- 2 cups of chicken or vegetable stock
- 1/2 cup dry white wine
- 1 head of radicchio that has been sliced into ribbons
- 1/4 cup of chopped chives
- 1 lemon zest and juice
- Olive oil
- flaky sea salt
- Parmigiano Reggiano cheese

<u>Cooking Directions</u>

- Rinse the soaked beans. Add the beans and a pinch of salt to a medium pot with a tablespoon of olive oil and sweat the shallots. After that, add the wine and cook until half of the liquid is gone. Pour in the chicken stock over the beans and heat to the point of boiling. Cover after it reaches a boiling point.

- After the beans have reached the desired al dente consistency, remove them from the stock and set them aside to cool. Add water and continue cooking the beans until they are cooked if the stock boils off before they are tender.
- In a large bowl, toss the beans and radicchio together. Toss in the lemon zest and a fresh squeeze of lemon before adding the olive oil and chives. Sliver of parmigiano reggiano cheese, flaky sea salt, and freshly ground pepper are the garnishes.

Carrot turmeric hummus

Ingredients

- 2 cups chopped carrots
- 1 clove of garlic
- 1 teaspoon grated fresh turmeric
- 2 lemons
- one-half cup extra-virgin olive oil
- additional ingredients for serving
- freshly ground black pepper and sea salt
- 2 tablespoons toasted,
- 2 tablespoons unsalted, hulled sunflower seeds
- Sumac
- vegetable crudités, for serving: sliced fresh mint leaves

Cooking Directions

- Ice and water should be added to a large bowl.
- In a small pot, bring some water to a boil.

- Cook the carrots until crisp-tender by adding them.
- Transfer immediately to the ice water after draining. At the point when cool, channel once more.
- Add the garlic, turmeric, lemon zest and juice, and ¼ cup water to the 7-cup KitchenAid Food Processor with the carrots. Blend till smooth.
- Add the olive oil in a constant flow while the machine is running. Add salt and pepper to taste.
- Top with the mint and sunflower seeds in a serving bowl.
- Zing the excess lemon straightforwardly on top, shower with olive oil, and sprinkle with sumac.
- Serve with bread crumbs.

Shredded kale and cranberry salad

<u>Ingredients</u>
- 1 block extra-firm tofu
- 1 head wavy kale
- 1 cup blended new spices, cleaved (I like to utilise mint, basil, and cilantro)
- 5 green onions, daintily cut
- 1/2 seedless cucumber, cut
- 1/2 cup dried cranberries
- 1/2 cup slashed peanuts
- 2 tablespoons olive oil, isolated
- 1 tablespoon soy sauce or tamari
- 2 teaspoons cornstarch
- fit salt and newly ground dark pepper

<u>For the citrus-ginger dressing:</u>
- Orange juice and zest

- ¼ cup olive oil
- 1 tablespoon soy sauce or tamari
- 1 tablespoon grated ginger
- 1 tablespoon honey
- 1 clove garlic
- 1 tablespoon rice vinegar
- a pinch of salt

Cooking Directions

- Dress the salad: consolidate all fixings in a blender and mix on medium until joined. Up to a week can be stored in a mason jar.
- Press the tofu: Slice your tofu into 1-inch pieces after removing it from its packaging and drying it off with paper towels. After placing them on a baking sheet or plate lined with paper towels, add two more layers of paper towels on top.
- To make it as heavy as possible, place your largest pan on top of it. Here, cast-iron works great. On the other hand, you can finish off it with a spot and a couple weighty jars to weigh it down. Allow it to sit for close to 30 minutes.
- Prep the kale in the meantime: After removing the tough ribs from the kale leaves, stack the leaves and slice them into ribbons.
- A teaspoon of extra-virgin olive oil should be drizzled over the kale in a large salad bowl. Massage the kale with both hands for about a minute until it becomes silky sweet and bright green and shrinks in size.
- Add 1 cup of high temp water to a bowl, then, at that point, add your cranberries. For them to become juicy and plump, let them sit for at least 15 minutes.

- How to cook tofu: It is dry and ready for searing after being pressed for 30 minutes. I prefer to cut the tofu into cubes at this point to create a "croutons"-like shape.
- Heat 1 tablespoon of oil in a skillet. Toss tofu with 1 teaspoon oil, tamari, and cornstarch in a bowl. Add to the pan, and cook until golden on one side. After carefully removing the tofu from the pan, cook it until golden brown and crispy on all sides, stirring occasionally. Toss the tofu in the pan with a little dressing, stir to coat, and then turn off the heat.
- Put the salad together: To the kale, add spices, green onions, cucumber, cranberries, peanuts, and tofu. Sprinkle with kosher salt and pepper to taste before tossing everything together until the dressing is evenly distributed. Eat!

Chapter Eight

Bread

Tender buckwheat bread

<u>Ingredients</u>
- 1¾ cups gluten-free all-purpose flour
- 1 teaspoon xanthan gum
- ½ cup buckwheat flour
- ¼ cup psyllium husk powder
- 1 teaspoon baking powder
- 2¼ teaspoons instant yeast
- 2 tablespoons of sugar

- 1 teaspoon salt
- ¼ cup vegetable oil
- 1 teaspoon apple cider vinegar
- 1½ cups warm water (approximately) 105 to 110 degrees Fahrenheit)
- 2 large, room-temperature eggs beaten

Cooking Directions

- Oil and Preheat: Oil a 9-by-4-inch nonstick metal loaf pan and preheat the oven to 350°F. Position the middle oven rack.
- Mix dry ingredients together: The gluten-free all-purpose flour, buckwheat flour, psyllium husk, baking powder, salt, instant yeast, and sugar are all combined in a large mixing bowl.
- Include Wet Components: Combine the warm water, apple cider vinegar, and vegetable oil thoroughly. The dough will be sticky and wet, but that's ok. Add the beaten eggs and mix for another minute until it resembles thick cake batter.
- Put the dough in the pan: Move the batter to the pre-arranged portion container and smooth out the top with a wet spatula.
- Dough Should Rise: In a warm, draft-free area, cover the pan with a kitchen towel and let it rise for another 30 minutes until it has roughly doubled in size.
- Bake: Heat for 40 to 50 minutes until the bread is dim brown on top and sounds empty when tapped.
- Completely cool: Before removing the loaf from the pan and cooling completely on a wire rack, allow it to cool for at least 10 minutes.
- Enjoy the Slice: After the bread has completely cooled, slice it with a serrated knife and enjoy!

Soft brown rice bread

<u>Ingredients</u>

- 2 cups brown rice flour
- 1¾ cups warm water (approximately 105-115 degrees Fahrenheit)
- ¼ cup sunflower oil
- ¼ cup psyllium husk powder
- 1 tablespoon instant yeast
- 2 tablespoons sugar
- ¾ teaspoon xanthan gum
- 2 eggs at room temperature
- 1 teaspoon baking powder
- ½ teaspoon salt

<u>Cooking Directions</u>

- Grease: Grease a loaf pan made of metal that measures 8 inches by 4 inches.
- Mix dry ingredients together: Brown rice flour, psyllium husk powder, instant yeast, sugar, baking powder, xanthan gum, and salt are all combined in a large mixing bowl.
- Add Fluid Fixings: Mix the dry ingredients well with the warm water, sunflower oil, and eggs to make a wet, shaggy dough (the dough is supposed to be shaggy, so don't worry).
- Put in the Pan: Smooth the top of the dough with a spatula after transferring it to the greased loaf pan.
- Dough Should Rise: Cover the batter skillet with a kitchen towel and let the mixture rise roughly 30 to 40 minutes in a warm, sans draft place until it has nearly multiplied in size.
- Turn on the oven: Preheat the oven to 350 degrees Fahrenheit and move the oven rack to the middle position during the dough's final ten minutes of rising.

- Bake: The dough should be baked for 40 to 50 minutes, or until the top of the loaf is dark brown and the loaf sounds hollow when tapped. Eliminate portion from the broiler.
- Completely cool: Allow the portion to cool for 10 minutes in the portion dish, prior to eliminating and allowing it to cool totally on the wire rack. After the loaf has fully cooled, slice it with a serrated knife.

Mashed potato bread

<u>Ingredients</u>

- 1 cup mashed potatoes
- 2 large beaten eggs
- 1 cup of warm water (between 105 and 115 degrees Fahrenheit)
- ¼ cup sunflower oil
- 2¼ cups gluten-free all-purpose flour
- 1 teaspoon xanthan gum
- 2 tablespoons psyllium husk powder
- 2¼ teaspoons instant yeast
- 1 tablespoon sugar
- ¼ teaspoon salt

<u>Cooking Directions</u>

- Grease: Use oil to grease an 8-by-4-inch loaf pan.

- Mix dry ingredients together: Sift the psyllium husk powder, instant yeast, gluten-free all-purpose flour, sugar, and salt into a large bowl. Mix well with a whisk.
- Blend: In a high-speed blender, combine the mashed potatoes and eggs to make a yellow, thick, and creamy mixture.
- Add oil and water: Place the ingredients in a large mixing bowl. A pale yellow liquid is produced when oil and water are combined well.
- Form the Pudding: Mix well the dry ingredients into the wet ingredients in the bowl until you have a uniform, sticky dough (the dough will look shaggy and be a little wet, but that's how you want it to feel).
- Put the dough in the pan: Smooth the dough's top with a wet spatula after transferring it to the prepared loaf pan.
- Let It Be: Place a kitchen towel over the pan and let the dough rise for 40 to 50 minutes in a warm, draft-free area until it has roughly doubled in size (I like to microwave the pan with the microwave off).
- Turn on the oven: While the mixture is rising, preheat the broiler to 350F and place the rack in the middle position.
- Prepare Until Brilliant Brown: Heat for 1 hour until the highest point of the bread is brilliant brown; the portion sounds empty when tapped.
- After cooling, slice: Before slicing, remove the loaf from the pan and place it on a wire rack to cool completely (at least 30 minutes) for 10 minutes.

Sorghum bread

<u>Ingredients</u>

- 1¾ cups gluten-free all-purpose flour
- 1 teaspoon xanthan gum
- ½ cup sorghum flour,
- 2 tablespoons psyllium husk powder
- 1 teaspoon baking powder
- 2 ¼ teaspoons instant yeast
- 2 tablespoons granulated white sugar
- 1 teaspoon salt
- ⅓ cup sunflower oil
- 1 teaspoon apple cider vinegar
- 1½ cups warm water, 105-115 degrees Fahrenheit
- 2 large eggs

<u>Cooking Directions</u>

- Butter the Pan: Grease a loaf pan made of metal that measures 8 inches by 4 inches.
- Mix dry ingredients together: Mix the gluten-free all-purpose flour, sorghum flour, psyllium husk powder, baking powder, salt, instant yeast, and sugar in a large mixing bowl until well combined.
- Include Wet Components: Warm water, eggs, sunflower oil, and apple cider vinegar should be added. The dough will be sticky and wet, but that is completely normal for gluten-free bread dough. Combine thoroughly for a few minutes until it resembles thick cake batter.
- Put the dough in the pan: Place the bread dough in the loaf pan that was previously greased, and smooth the top with a wet spatula.

- Dough Should Rise: In a warm, draft-free area, cover the pan with a kitchen towel and let the dough rise for 30 to 40 minutes, or until it has roughly doubled in size.
- Turn on the oven: Preheat the oven to 350°F and position the middle rack of the oven while the dough rises.
- Bake until brown and crispy: Bake the dough for 40 to 50 minutes in a preheated oven until it has doubled in size and the top is golden brown and the bread sounds hollow when tapped.
- Allow complete cooling: Before removing the loaf from the pan, let it cool for ten minutes on a wire rack before slicing it with a ridged knife.

Teff bread

<u>Ingredients</u>

- 1¾ cup without gluten regular flour
- 1 teaspoon thickener
- ½ cup teff flour
- 2 tablespoons psyllium husk powder
- 1 teaspoon baking powder
- 2 1/4 teaspoons moment yeast
- 2 tablespoons sugar
- 1 teaspoon salt
- ⅓ cup sunflower oil
- 1 teaspoon apple juice vinegar
- 1½ cups warm water (approx. 105 to 115 degrees Fahrenheit)

- 2 large, room-temperature eggs beaten

<u>Cooking Directions</u>
- Oil and Preheat: Preheat the broiler to 350F and organise the stove rack to the centre third position. Oil a nonstick metal loaf pan that is 8 inches by 4 inches.
- Mix dry ingredients together: Mix together the instant yeast, sugar, salt, gluten-free all-purpose flour, psyllium husk powder, teff flour, xanthan gum (if using), and baking powder in a large mixing bowl.
- Include Wet Components: Combine the warm water, apple cider vinegar, and vegetable oil thoroughly. The mixture will be sticky and wet, yet that is the very surface you need. Add the beaten eggs and mix for another minute until it looks like thick cake batter.
- Put the dough in the pan: Move the teff bread mixture to the pre-arranged portion container and smooth out the top with a wet spatula.
- Dough Should Rise: Cover the dish with a kitchen towel and let the batter rise for around 30 to 40 minutes in a warm, sans draft place, until it has generally multiplied in size. (Tip: While the dough rises, I prefer to place the pan in the microwave with the microwave off.)
- Bake until finished: Teff bread should be baked for 50 to 60 minutes, or until it sounds hollow when tapped and has a dark brown top.
- Completely cool: Before removing the loaf from the pan and cooling it completely on a wire rack, allow it to cool for at least 10 minutes.

Whole grain bread

<u>Ingredients</u>

- ¾ cup brown rice flour
- ¾ cup sorghum flour
- ½ cup millet flour
- ⅓ cup potato starch
- ⅓ cup tapioca starch
- 1 teaspoon xanthan gum
- 1 teaspoon baking powder
- 1½ teaspoons salt
- 2 tablespoons psyllium husk powder
- 2¼ teaspoons instant yeast
- 2 tablespoons sugar
- 1½ cups warm water
- ⅓ cup sunflower oil

<u>Cooking Directions</u>

- Oil the loaf pan: Grease a loaf pan made of nonstick metal that measures 8 inches by 4 inches.
- Mix dry ingredients together: Brown rice flour, sorghum flour, millet flour, potato starch, tapioca starch, xanthan gum, baking powder, salt, psyllium husk powder, instant yeast, and sugar are all combined in a large mixing bowl. Mix well with a whisk.
- Add Wet Fixings to Frame Batter: To make a uniform, wet, and sticky dough, combine the dry ingredients in a large bowl with the warm water and vegetable oil.
- Move Batter to Portion Skillet: Move the sans gluten entire grain bread mixture to the recently lubed portion dish and smooth out the highest point of the batter with a wet spatula.

- Allow Mixture To rise: The dough should be allowed to rise for one hour in a warm, draft-free location until it has nearly doubled in size and risen to the top of the pan.
- Turn on the oven: Preheat the oven to 350F in the final 15 minutes of the rise and position the middle oven rack.
- Prepare Until Brilliant: Bake the dough until it is golden brown and a hollow sound is made when tapped on the loaf.
- Before slicing, let it cool completely: Before slicing the gluten-free whole grain loaf, allow it to completely cool on a wire rack at room temperature.

Pumpkin yeast bread

<u>Ingredients</u>

- 1 cup pumpkin puree
- 2 large, beaten eggs
- 1 cup of warm water (between 105 and 115 degrees Fahrenheit)
- ¼ cup sunflower oil
- 2¾ cups gluten-free all-purpose flour
- 1 teaspoon of xanthan gum
- 2 tablespoons psyllium husk powder
- 2¼ teaspoons instant yeast
- 1 tablespoon sugar
- 1 teaspoon baking powder
- ¼ teaspoon salt

<u>Cooking Directions</u>

- Oil the loaf pan: Oil a 8″ x 4″ metal portion skillet.
- Whisk Dry Fixings: In a huge bowl, filter the sans gluten regular flour, thickener (if utilising), psyllium husk powder, moment yeast, sugar, baking powder and salt. Whisk well to consolidate.
- Process the eggs and pumpkin: Consolidate the pumpkin puree and eggs in the bowl of a high velocity blender or food processor and cycle until you get a thick rich orange combination.
- Add oil and water: Add oil and water to a large mixing bowl with the pumpkin-egg mixture. To create an orange liquid mixture, thoroughly mix.
- To make dough, add dry ingredients like: Add the dry fixings to the bowl with the wet fixings and blend well to get a tacky mixture (the pumpkin yeast bread batter will be shaggy and wet, and that is unequivocally the way in which it ought to be).
- Move Batter to Portion Dish: Move the mixture to the recently lubed portion container and smooth out the highest point of the batter with a wet spatula.
- Allow Mixture To rise: The dough should rise for 40 to 50 minutes in a warm, wind-free area until it has roughly doubled in size.
- Turn on the oven: Preheat the oven to 350°F (180°C) and position the middle baking rack while the dough is almost ready to rise.
- Bake to a golden colour: Bake for one hour, or until the top is golden brown and the loaf sounds hollow when tapped, after the dough has finished rising.
- After cooling, slice: Before slicing the loaf, let it cool completely to room temperature on a wire rack.

Pumpernickel bread

<u>Ingredients</u>

- 1½ cups sans gluten regular flour
- ¾ teaspoon thickener
- ¾ cups teff flour
- 2 tablespoons psyllium husk powder
- ¼ cup unsweetened cocoa powder
- 1 teaspoon baking powder
- 2¼ teaspoons moment yeast
- 1 tablespoon sugar
- 1 teaspoon salt
- ¼ cup molasses
- ⅓ cup sunflower oil
- 1 teaspoon vinegar
- 1⅓ cups warm water (between 105F to 115F)
- 2 large eggs, beaten

<u>Cooking Directions</u>

- Preheat and Lube: Oil a 8″ x 4″ metal portion skillet and afterward preheat the broiler to 350F. Orchestrate the stove rack to the centre position.
- Consolidate Dry Fixings: In a huge blending bowl, join the without gluten regular flour, thickener (teff flour, psyllium husk powder, unsweetened cocoa powder, baking powder, moment yeast, sugar and salt. Whisk well to consolidate.
- Add Wet Fixings: Add the molasses, sunflower oil, vinegar, warm water, and beaten eggs to the huge bowl with the dry fixings. Blend well until you get a wet, tacky mixture that looks like earthy coloured cake hitter.

- Move to Portion Dish: Move the pumpernickel bread batter to the beforehand lubed portion container and smooth out the top with a wet spatula.
- Let Rise: Let the mixture ascend in a warm, without draft place for no less than 30 minutes until it has multiplied in size.
- Prepare Until Prepared: Heat the mixture for 50 to an hour until the portion is dim brown on top and sounds empty when tapped.
- Cool Completely: Permit the without gluten pumpernickel portion to cool for no less than 10 minutes in the portion dish prior to eliminating it and allowing it to cool totally at room temperature on a wire rack.
- Cut and Appreciate: When the portion has completely cooled, cut and appreciate!

Cheeseburger buns

<u>Ingredients</u>

- 2¼ cups sans gluten regular flour
- ¾ teaspoon thickener
- 1 teaspoon baking powder
- 1 teaspoon salt
- 2¼ teaspoons moment yeast
- 1 tablespoons sugar
- 2 tablespoons psyllium husk powder
- ⅓ cup sunflower oil + something else for brushing
- 1 teaspoon white vinegar (or apple juice vinegar)
- 1½ cups warm water
- 2 enormous eggs, beaten, room temperature
- 2 tablespoons white sesame seeds

<u>Cooking Directions</u>

- Preheat, Line and Oil: Preheat broiler to 350F and line an enormous baking sheet with material paper or a silpat. Oil 6 round metal rings and put on the mat.
- Whisk Dry Fixings: In an enormous blending bowl, whisk the sans gluten regular flour, thickener (if utilising), baking powder, salt, moment yeast, sugar and psyllium husk powder.
- Add Wet Fixings: Add the vegetable oil, vinegar, warm water and beaten eggs. Blend well until you get a mixture that looks like a cake player (the batter will be shaggy and wet, however that is the consistency you need).
- Split Mixture Between Rings: Gap the batter equally between the metal rings and smooth out the highest points of the mixture with the rear of a wet spoon.
- Let Ascend Until Multiplied: Permit the batter ascend in a warm, without draft place until it has generally multiplied in size. (Contingent upon the temperature and dampness, it might require just 30 minutes in a warm and moist environment or as long as 1 hour in the colder time of year).
- Brush with Oil: Utilise a silicon brush to brush the highest points of the batter with oil.
- Sprinkle Seeds on Top: Sprinkle sesame seeds on top of the mixture.
- Heat: Prepare the buns for 30 to 40 minutes until browns on top.
- Let Cool Prior to Eliminating: When heated, let the sans gluten burger buns cool for no less than 10 minutes in the rings prior to eliminating them to cool totally at room temperature on a wire rack.

Chapter Nine

Dinner

Chicken fajita marinade

<u>Ingredients</u>
For the marinade

- 1/4 cup soy sauce use sans gluten if necessary
- 2 tablespoons oil
- 1/4 cup earthy coloured sugar
- 2 tablespoons lime juice
- 2 tablespoons white vinegar
- 3 cloves garlic minced

- 1 teaspoon salt
- 1/4 teaspoon ground ginger
- 1/2 teaspoon pepper
- 1 teaspoon bean stew powder
- 1 teaspoon cumin

For the fajitas

- 3 boneless skinless chicken bosoms, cut into slight strips
- 1/2 enormous red onion daintily cut
- 1 medium green pepper meagerly cut
- 1 medium red pepper meagerly cut
- 2 medium tomatoes cleaved (discretionary)
- Guidelines

<u>Cooking Directions</u>

- Blend every one of the elements for the marinate together in an enormous ziploc sack or shallow dish. Add the cut chicken and blend to equitably cover it. Marinate for somewhere around 1 hour or as long as 12 hours.
- Heat an enormous skillet with 1 tablespoon of oil. Add the chicken and all the marinade to the skillet and saute for 3-4 minutes, carrying the sauce to a full bubble.
- Add the cut onions, peppers, and tomatoes and cook until they are simply delicate, another 5-7 minutes.
- Serve on corn tortillas with your #1 fixings like avocado, feta cheddar (or queso fresco), and salsa. Appreciate!

Instant Pot BBQ Chicken

<u>Ingredients</u>

- 1 cup chicken stock or water
- 2 lbs chicken thighs
- 1 lb chicken bosom
- 1/2 teaspoon onion powder
- 1/2 teaspoon garlic powder
- 1/2 teaspoon paprika
- 1/2 teaspoon salt
- 1 1/2 cups bar-b-que sauce
- 1/2 cup ground onion in addition to juice
- 2-3 tablespoons earthy coloured sugar
- 2 teaspoons Worcestershire sauce

<u>Cooking Directions</u>

- Place the fixings in the moment pot in a specific order: chicken stock (or water), chicken, onion powder, garlic, powder, paprika, salt, bar-b-que sauce, ground onion, earthy coloured sugar and Worcestershire sauce. Try not to mix. You believe the water should remain on the lower part of the pot so the moment the pot comes to pressure.
- Put the top on the moment pot ensuring the valve is in the fixing position. Press manual (high tension) and set to 15 minutes. Allow the tension normally to deliver for 10 minutes. Then, at that point, quickly deliver the venting position to deliver the excess tension and open the pot.
- Eliminate the chicken and shred it. In the event that is important, lessen the fluid by squeezing the "saute" button and stewing the

sauce, blending frequently, until thickened. Add the chicken back to the sauce prior to serving.

- Add more bar-b-que sauce whenever wanted. Shred and appreciated on sandwiches, mixed greens, bar-b-que plates from there,

Gluten free enchiladas

<u>Ingredients</u>
<u>For the red sauce</u>

- 1 medium onion diced
- 1 jalapeño cultivated and cleaved
- 1 tablespoon oil
- 3 medium cloves garlic finely minced
- 2 tablespoons stew powder
- 1 tablespoon earthy coloured sugar
- 2 teaspoons ground cumin
- ½ teaspoon oregano
- ½ teaspoon salt
- 15 oz might tomato at any point sauce
- 1 cup chicken or vegetable stock

<u>For the Chicken Filling</u>

- 1-11/2 lbs boneless skinless chicken bosoms (2-3 large bosoms)
- 1 1/2 cups (6 ounces) sharp cheddar newly destroyed
- 1 1/2 cups (6 ounces) Monterey jack cheddar newly destroyed
- 1/2 cup new cilantro minced
- 1 lime

- 12 6-inch delicate corn tortillas

<u>Cooking Directions</u>

Make the sauce

- In a huge pot, add the onion, jalapeno and oil. Cook on medium intensity until the vegetables have mellowed, 8-10 minutes.
- Mix in the garlic, stew powder, cumin, oregano, sugar and salt and cook until fragrant, 30 seconds to 1 moment. Add the pureed tomatoes and chicken stock and mix to consolidate. Settle in the chicken. Carry the blend to a stew.
- Diminish intensity to low and stew for 15 minutes until the sauce has thickened somewhat. Eliminate the chicken and spot in a bowl. (Discretionary however suggested: Cautiously empty the sauce into a blender and mix until smooth.) Season the sauce with a touch more salt, if important and put away.

<u>Make the filling</u>

- Preheat the broiler to 400F. Softly oil a 9×13 baking dish.
- Shred the chicken into reduced down pieces. Add 1 cup of the sharp cheddar, 1 cup of the Monterey jack cheddar, the cilantro and the juice of 1 lime to the chicken. Blend to join. (Put away the remainder of the cheddar for garnish the enchiladas.)
- Stack the tortillas on a plate and cover with cling wrap or moist paper towels. Microwave on high until warm and flexible, 20-30 seconds.
- Scoop 1/3 cup of the chicken blend on top of a tortilla and press it equally down the centre. (You'll partition the filling to make 12 enchiladas.) Firmly roll every tortilla and lay the crease side down in the baking dish. Rehash with the excess tortillas.
- Pour the sauce over the enchiladas and top with the leftover cheddar. Cover the baking dish firmly with foil. Heat covered for 20-25 minutes. Eliminate the foil and keep on baking for

another 5-10 minutes until brilliant and effervescent. Eliminate from the broiler and let it represent 10 minutes prior to serving.

Gluten-free Chicken Potpie

Ingredients

- 1 3/4 cups sans gluten 1:1 baking flour
- 4 teaspoons baking powder
- 1/2 teaspoon salt
- 1 tablespoon sugar
- 1 cup milk
- 1 egg whisked
- 3 tablespoons margarine softened

For the egg wash

- 1 egg
- 1 tablespoon water
- For the chicken pot pie:
- ¼ cup gluten-free all purpose flour
- ¼ cup butter
- 1 medium yellow onion diced
- ¾ teaspoon sal
- ¾ teaspoon ground pepper
- 1 teaspoon smoked paprika
- ¼ teaspoon ground mustard
- ⅛ teaspoon dried thyme
- 3 cups chicken stock
- ½ cup heavy cream
- 3 cups diced peeled russet potatoes

- 2 carrots chopped,
- 3 cups frozen mixed vegetables,

<u>Cooking Directions</u>
<u>Pre-bake the biscuit</u>
- Line a baking sheet with parchment paper or a silicone baking mat and preheat the oven to 400 degrees Fahrenheit.
- In the bowl of a stand blender, add the sans gluten flour, baking powder, salt and sugar. Combine everything to combine. Mix in the butter, milk, and egg until well combined.
- Scoop eight large spoonfuls of the batter onto the baking sheet quickly. Smooth or form the scoop's top into a biscuit shape with wet fingers. Brush the tops of each biscuit with the egg wash that has been whisked together.
- Bake until set for ten minutes. Set aside while the filling is ready after removing it from the oven. The filling will complete the baking process.)

<u>Create the filling by:</u>
- Melt the butter in a large Dutch oven or pot over medium heat. Because this is the pot in which you will bake your pot pie, make sure it is big enough!
- Add the chopped onion and cook for 5-7 minutes until soft.
- Sprinkle the sans gluten flour over the onion combination and race until smooth. Combine the mustard and thyme with the salt, pepper, and paprika.
- Steadily mix in the chicken stock and weighty cream. Add the potatoes and carrots, and heat the blend to the point of boiling over medium intensity, mixing habitually until the fluid has thickened and the potatoes and carrots are delicate when penetrated with a fork, around 15-20 minutes. Add the frozen

vegetables and cook for an additional 5 to 10 minutes, or until they are tender.

<u>Bake the pie</u>

- Eliminate from the intensity and mix in the destroyed chicken. Bake the pre-baked biscuits on top of the gluten-free pot pie for 20 to 25 minutes, or until they begin to turn a light golden brown and are cooked through. Serve and have fun!

Slow cooker Moroccan chicken

<u>Ingredients</u>

For the chicken

- 3 tablespoons olive oil or avocado oil
- 2-3 pounds boneless skinless chicken thighs
- salt and pepper
- 1 onion meagerly cut
- 3 cloves garlic minced
- 3 tablespoons almond spread
- 3/4 cup chicken stock
- 1/2 teaspoon salt

All the other things:

- 1 teaspoon cumin
- 1/2 teaspoon ginger
- 1/2 teaspoon coriander
- 1/4 teaspoon cinnamon
- a pinch of cayenne pepper
- 1 pound baby carrots

- 1/2 cup dried apricots
- 1/4 cup dried cherries
- 1 teaspoon brown sugar or coconut sugar

<u>Cooking Directions</u>
- Salt and pepper season the chicken on both sides. Heat 1 tablespoon of olive oil in a huge skillet over medium-high intensity. Add half of the chicken thighs to the hot pan and cook for 3 to 4 minutes on each side. The chicken can be browned on the outside for flavour without being cooked through. After placing the chicken in the slow cooker, continue with the remaining thighs.
- Add the sliced onions to the empty skillet over medium heat. Cook for three to four minutes, scraping up any brown bits from the bottom of the pan. After being added, cook the garlic for 30 seconds.
- Scrape the pan's bottom after adding the chicken stock. Incorporate the salt, sugar, and spices with the almond butter.
- Transfer the mixture of onion and stock to the slow cooker. After mixing everything together, add the carrots. On low, cook for four hours.
- Add the apricots and cherries after 4 hours, and cook for another 1 to 2 hours.
- Serve the meat over cooked quinoa and lightly shred it. Enjoy!

Instant pot southwestern chicken and rice

<u>Ingredients</u>
- 1 1/2 cups brown rice
- 3/4 cup salsa

- 15 ounces kidney beans (drained and rinsed)
- 1/2 cup frozen corn
- 1 1/2 cups chicken stock
- 1 teaspoon chilli powder
- 1/2 teaspoon garlic powder
- 1/4 teaspoon cumin
- 1/2 teaspoon salt
- 2 chicken breasts
- 1/2 cup shredded sharp cheddar
- chips hot sauce and additional cheese for serving

<u>Cooking Directions</u>

- Place Mix thoroughly.
- Place the chicken breasts in the rice/liquid mixture, leaving them whole to prevent drying out during cooking. Sprinkle the bean stew powder, garlic powder, onion powder, cumin and salt part of the way over the chicken and incompletely over the fluid/rice combination. Spread the spices out and use a spoon to mix some of them in with the liquid. This does not need to be exact. Simply sprinkle some on the chicken and add some to the rice.
- Close the lid and cook for 24 minutes at HIGH PRESSURE Slowly release the remaining pressure after letting the pressure naturally release for ten minutes. Eliminate the chicken bosoms and shred into scaled down pieces. With a fork, mix the chicken and shredded cheese into the rice.
- Dip chips in hot sauce and cheese before serving. Enjoy!

Gluten-free chilli

<u>Ingredients</u>

- 1 tablespoon olive oil

- 1 pound ground beef
- 1 pound sausage
- 1 large onion chopped (about 2 cups)
- 1 green pepper chopped (about 1 cup)
- 1 jalapeno pepper seeded and minced
- 2 tablespoons chilli powder
- 1 tablespoon cumin
- 1 teaspoon oregano
- 1/2 teaspoon salt
- 1/4 teaspoon pepper
- 1 tablespoon brown sugar
- 2 bay leaves
- 4 cloves minced garlic
- 3 tablespoons tomato paste
- 2 28 oz cans crushed tomatoes

<u>Cooking Directions</u>

For the instant pot

- Select Saute from the Instant Pot menu. Olive oil must be added. Using a spatula or meat chopper to break up the beef and sausage as you stir, add the meat and cook until browned.
- Add the onion, green pepper and jalapeno and cook for 3 additional minutes or until mellowed.
- Cook for 1-2 minutes until fragrant before adding the chilli powder, cumin, oregano, salt, pepper, brown sugar, bay leaves, garlic, and tomato paste.
- Pour in the squashed tomatoes, chicken stock and beans and mix to consolidate. Cook for 15 minutes by selecting MANUAL or High Pressure on the instant pot. For ten minutes, allow the natural release of the chilli.

- Present with most loved fixings. Enjoy!

For the stove pot

- Heat a huge dutch broiler or pot over medium-high intensity. Olive oil must be added. Using a spatula or meat chopper to break up the beef and sausage as you stir, add the meat and cook until browned.
- Add the onion, green pepper and jalapeno and cook for 3 additional minutes or until mellowed.
- Cook for 1-2 minutes until fragrant before adding the chilli powder, cumin, oregano, salt, pepper, brown sugar, bay leaves, garlic, and tomato paste.
- Add the beans, chicken stock, and crushed tomatoes and stir to combine. Reduce the heat to a simmer, then cook for 40 to 50 minutes while stirring frequently. Before serving, let the mixture sit for ten minutes with the lid on and the heat off.
- Top with your preferred toppings. Enjoy!

Gluten-free beef stew

<u>Ingredients</u>

- 4 lbs hamburger stew meat 1-2 inch 3D squares
- 2 tablespoons olive oil
- 1 large onion halved and cut from pole to pole into 1/8-inch-thick slices (about 2 cups)
- 4 medium carrots that have been peeled and cut into 1-inch pieces
- 2 cloves of minced garlic
- 1 tablespoon tomato paste

- 2-3 tablespoons gluten-free flour
- 1 cup beef broth, 1 cup red wine
- 3 cups gluten-free low-sodium beef broth/stock
- 2 bay leaves
- 4 springs thyme
- 4 ounces salt, or pork trimmed of excess fat
- 1 pound yukon gold potatoes cut into 1 inch chunks
- 1 cup frozen peas

<u>Cooking Directions</u>

- In a Dutch oven, heat 1 tablespoon of olive oil over high heat until it shimmers. Cook the other half of the beef for about 8 minutes, or until well browned on all sides. If the fond or oil starts to smoke, turn down the heat. Move the beef over to the slow cooker.
- Add the remaining beef and one tablespoon of olive oil to the slow cooker in a second step.
- If necessary, add the onion and carrots to the empty Dutch oven with two teaspoons of olive oil. Cook, scratching the lower part of the container to slacken any seared pieces, until the onion is relaxed, 3-4 minutes.
- Add the flour and cook, blending continually, until no dry flour stays, around 30 seconds. Add garlic, tomato glue and cook, mixing continually, until fragrant, around 30 seconds.
- Gradually add the wine, scratching the lower part of the container to slacken any seared pieces. Increment intensity to high and permit wine to stew until thickened and marginally diminished, around 2 minutes. Blend in the beef broth.

- Empty the vegetable stock combination into the sluggish cooker. Add the salt pork, thyme, and bay leaves by stirring.
- Cook on low for 4-6 hours (or high for 3-4 hours). Remove the salt from the pork two hours before serving and add the potatoes.
- 30 minutes prior to eating the mix in the peas.

Sloppy joes

<u>Ingredients</u>

- 2 tablespoons olive oil
- 1 huge onion hacked
- 2 1/2 pounds ground meat or turkey
- 2/3 cup BBQ sauce be certain it is without gluten,
- 1/2 cup ketchup
- 1/4 cup tamari (without gluten soy sauce)
- 3 tablespoons Worcestershire sauce be certain it is without gluten
- 3 tablespoons tomato glue
- 1/2 teaspoon dark pepper
- 8 without gluten buns

<u>Cooking Directions</u>

- In a huge dutch stove over medium intensity, add the olive oil and cleaved onion. Saute until mellowed, around 5-7 minutes.

- Add the meat and cook, mixing and separating it until it is finely ground. Cook until caramelised, around 10 minutes. Channel the oil off the meat and vegetables.
- Mix in the bar-b-que sauce, ketchup, tamari, Worcestershire sauce, tomato glue, soy sauce and 1/2 teaspoon ground pepper. Stew for around 10-15 minutes, until thickened.
- Serve over toasted buns. Appreciate!

Alfredo sauce

<u>Ingredients</u>

- 3 tablespoons margarine
- 1 clove garlic finely minced
- 4 ounces cream cheddar cut into 1-inch solid shapes
- 1 cup milk ideally entire milk yet 2% will work
- 1 1/2 cups 3-6 ounces newly ground Parmesan cheddar
- 1/2 teaspoon salt
- 1/4 teaspoon pepper

<u>Cooking Directions</u>

- In a medium pot or skillet over medium intensity, liquefy the spread. Add the garlic and cook for around 1 moment, mixing continually so the garlic doesn't consume.
- Add the cream cheddar to the spread combination and allow it to sit for a couple of moments until it starts to liquefy. Whisk the margarine and cream cheddar together until smooth and velvety.

This might require a couple of moments of racing to get thoroughly smooth.

- While whisking, gradually add the milk a little at once and integrate. Mix in the Parmesan cheddar, salt and pepper. Blend until everything is smooth and consolidated.
- Cook for 2-3 minutes for a thicker sauce or eliminate just after the cheddar is softened for a more slender sauce. If necessary, add more salt and pepper to taste. Serve promptly over sans gluten pasta.

Lasagna

<u>Ingredients</u>
<u>For the Cheddar Combination:</u>

- 1 16 oz pack of destroyed mozzarella cheddar low-dampness
- 8 oz ricotta cheddar
- 8oz curds little curd
- 1/2 cup ground parmesan cheddar
- 2 eggs
- 1 teaspoon dried parsley
- 1/2 teaspoon pepper

For the sauce

- 1 lb ground hamburger
- 1/2 white onion finely diced
- 29 oz can Chase's Pureed tomatoes or one more canned pureed tomatoes

- 24-28 oz bottle bumped tomato basil pasta sauce I like the Tomato Basil sauce from Broker Joe's ideal
- 10oz Sans gluten Broiler Prepared Lasagna Noodles

Cooking Directions

- Preheat the stove to 425F.
- Put away one cup of the mozzarella cheddar for fixing the lasagna later. In a medium bowl, combine as one the leftover mozzarella and rest of the cheddar blend fixings until joined.
- In a huge skillet over medium-high intensity, add the ground hamburger and onion. Brown the ground meat, breaking into tiny lumps as you do. (The more modest the better so there aren't huge lumps of meat in the lasagna.)
- Channel the meat of any abundance of oil and return to the container. Add the sauces and blend until warmed through.
- Spoon a meagre layer of sauce onto the lower part of a 9×13 baking dish. Involving 5 noodles for the main layer - plunge a noodle in the sauce and spread the highest point of the noodle with a layer of sauce. Place in the dish. Plunging/covering every individual noodle with sauce guarantees the noodles will cook through. (See the photographs in the post.) Rehash with the leftover noodles. You might need to break the fifth noodle in half to fit it along the lower part of the skillet. Assuming that it breaks no issue, simply layer it in all that can be expected!
- Layer the remainder of the lasagna as follows:Add 1/2 of the cheddar blend in spots across the highest point of the noodle/sauce layer. Spread with a little spatula until smooth. Spread a couple of little spoonfuls of sauce over the cheddar layer. Plunge/cover one more 5 noodles and lay them on top of the cheddar combination. Add the other 1/2 of the cheddar blend

in bits across the highest point of the noodle/sauce layer. Spread with a little spatula until smooth.Spread a couple of little spoonfuls of sauce over the cheddar layer.Dip/cover the leftover 6 noodles in sauce and lay them on top. Spread any excess sauce over top of the lasagna.

- Cover the dish firmly with aluminium foil. Prepare for 40 minutes covered. Eliminate the foil and top with the saved mozzarella cheddar. Heat for another 15-20 minutes until seared and gurgling.
- Before serving, let the lasagna sit for 20 minutes. Cut and appreciate

Sweetcorn soup

<u>Ingredients</u>

- 1 tablespoon olive oil
- 1 little red-cleaned potato stripped and slashed
- 1 little carrot slashed (1/3 cup)
- 1 little onion slashed (1/3 cup)
- 1 clove garlic minced
- 4 cups chicken stock
- 6 cups corn new or frozen
- salt and pepper
- 2-3 tablespoons new parsley or thyme
- 2 limes
- hot sauce or margarine

<u>Cooking Directions</u>

- Heat a medium/enormous pot over medium intensity. Add the olive oil alongside the potato, carrot and onion. Cook until the onion is delicate, around 6-7 minutes. Cook the garlic for 30 seconds after adding it.
- Pour in the chicken stock and mix. Add salt and pepper - around 1/4 to 1/2 teaspoon each relying upon pungency of your stock. Heat to the point of boiling then, at that point, cover and diminish to a stew for 5 minutes.
- Cover and cook for 10 to 15 minutes, or until the vegetables are tender, adding 3 cups of corn. Move the combination to a blender and mix until smooth. On the other hand you can use a drenching blender to mix until smooth.
- Empty the soup once again into the pot. Add the leftover 3 cups corn, parsley and salt and pepper to taste. Present with a crush of lime and margarine/hot sauce. Appreciate!

Chapter Ten

Dessert

Flourless chocolate pecan treats

<u>Ingredients</u>

- 3 c. confectioners' sugar
- 3/4 c. Dutch-handled cocoa powder
- 1/2 tsp. genuine salt
- 2 large eggs, at room temp
- 1 tsp. unadulterated vanilla concentrate
- 1 c. toasted pecans, slashed
- 1/2 c. clashing or dim chocolate chips
- Flaky ocean salt

<u>Cooking Directions</u>

- Heat broiler to 350°F. Line 2 baking sheets with material paper and gently cover with cooking shower.
- Whisk together sugar, cocoa powder, and salt in a medium bowl. Utilising an electric blender, beat together eggs and vanilla. Add sugar combination and blend to join; overlay in pecans and chocolate chips.
- Spoon player (around 1 1/2 Tbsp per treat) onto arranged baking sheets, separating 2 in. separated, and sprinkle with flaky ocean salt.
- Bake, pivoting places of dish once, until treats are puffed and beat start to break, 12 to 14 minutes. Let cool on baking sheets for 5 minutes, then slide material and treats to wire racks to totally cool.

Vegan apple cake

<u>Ingredients</u>

For Cake

- 7 1/2 c. almond flour
- 1 1/2 c. potato starch
- 1/2 c. cornstarch
- 2 c. granulated sugar
- 3 tsp. ground cinnamon
- 2 1/4 tsp. baking powder
- 2 1/4 tsp. baking pop
- 1 1/2 tsp. ground allspice
- 1 1/2 tsp. ground ginger
- 3/4 tsp. ground nutmeg
- 1/2 tsp. legitimate salt
- 2 1/2 c. oat milk or other dairy free milk
- 2 1/4 tsp. juice vinegar
- 3 tbsp. unsulphured molasses
- 1 1/2 tsp. unadulterated vanilla concentrate
- 1/2 c. unsweetened fruit purée

For Icing

- 3 c. apple juice
- 1 lb. veggie lover margarine
- 1 lb. confectioners' sugar, filtered

<u>Cooking Directions</u>

- Prepare cake: Intensity stove to 350°F. Delicately cover three 8-inch cake skillets with non-stick cooking splash. Line bottoms with material; shower material. In an enormous bowl, consolidate almond flour, potato starch, cornstarch, granulated sugar, cinnamon, baking powder, baking pop, allspice, ginger, nutmeg, and salt.

- In a subsequent bowl, join oat milk, vinegar, molasses, and vanilla. Overlay into flour combination, then, at that point, overlap in fruit purée.
- Evenly split the batter between pre-arranged containers (around 2 1/3 cups in each dish), spread equitably, and heat until brilliant brown and toothpick embedded into the middle confesses all, 30 to 35 minutes. Allow cakes to cool totally in the dish.
- Meanwhile get ready icing: In a little pot, stew apple juice until decreased to around 2 tablespoons, 30 to 35 minutes. Let cool. While juice syrup is cooling, eliminate vegetarian spread from the cooler and let sit at room temperature for 20 minutes yet don't permit it to get excessively delicate (return to the fridge momentarily on the off chance that this occurs).
- Using an electric blender on medium speed, beat veggie lover margarine, confectioners' sugar, and decreased juice until smooth and cushy, around 4 minutes. Makes around 4 1/2 cups icing. (Assuming it is excessively delicate, return to the fridge to solidify.)
- Place one cake layer, base side up, on a serving plate and spread piling 1/2 cup frosting uniformly up and over. Top with another cake, base side up; rehash. Spread excess frosting up and over the sides of the cake.

Ice cream float

Ingredients

- 3 tbsp. soft drink syrup or mixed drink syrup
- 2 tbsp. creamer
- Club pop
- Vanilla frozen yoghurt
- Whipped cream, for serving (discretionary)

<u>Cooking Directions</u>
- In a tall glass, mix together syrup and creamer. Add sufficient club pop so it comes around 3/4 up the glass. Add 2 scoops of frozen yoghurt and top with whipped cream whenever wanted.

Sea salted nut butter cups

<u>Ingredients</u>
- 1 ready medium banana
- 1/4 c. nut margarine
- 12 oz. self-contradicting chocolate
- Flaky ocean salt, for sprinkling

<u>Cooking Directions</u>
- Line 2 is a smaller than usual biscuit container with foil liners.
- In a little bowl, pound banana with nut margarine.
- Place chocolate in a second bowl. Microwave on high for 30 seconds at a time, stirring between each interval, until smooth and melted.
- Drop a scant teaspoon of chocolate into each liner, then spoon 1 teaspoon nut-butter mixture on top. Spread enough chocolate to cover the surface.
- Sprinkle each with ocean salt and freeze until firm.

Molten chocolate skillet brownies

<u>Ingredients</u>

- 1 stick (1/2 cup) chopped butter
- 8 ounces finely chopped dark chocolate
- 4 four large, separated eggs
- 2 tablespoons unsweetened cocoa
- 1 tsp. salt
- 1/4 teaspoon vanilla extract
- 2/3 c. sugar
- Raspberries and vanilla frozen yoghurt yogurt, for serving

Cooking Directions

- Preheat the broiler to 350°F. Grease four miniature cast-iron skillets measuring 6 to 6.5 inches; place on an enormous baking sheet. Microwave the chocolate and butter in a large microwave-safe bowl for 30 seconds on high until the chocolate has melted, stirring in between. Blend the mixture by stirring; place aside.

- In a medium bowl, whisk egg yolks, cocoa, vanilla, salt and a big part of sugar until smooth; incorporate with the chocolate mixture. In another bowl, with a blender on medium-rapid, beat egg whites until they have a delicate pinnacles structure. Beat in the rest of the sugar until stiff peaks form.

- thoroughly combine the chocolate mixture with one-fourth of the beaten whites. Gently fold the remaining whites into the chocolate mixture in two batches without deflating the whites.

Split player between skillets; Place in the oven. Puffed, baked for 15 to 18 minutes. Serve warm with berries and ice cream after 10 minutes of standing

Roasted strawberries

<u>Ingredients</u>

- 1 lb. strawberries, cut in half or in quarters if large,
- 2 tablespoons Warm honey
- Kosher salt
- half a vanilla bean.

<u>Cooking Directions</u>

- The first step is to heat the oven to 350°F. Leave a 1-inch overhang on two long sides of a 9-by-13-inch baking pan that has been lined with parchment.
- Toss the strawberries with honey and a pinch of salt in the pan that has been prepared. Split the vanilla bean in half lengthwise. Add the seeds and scraped pod to the strawberry mixture and toss to combine.
- Roast for 40 to 50 minutes, stirring once, until the strawberries are tender and the juices start to reduce but not brown.

Keto almond butter fudge

<u>Ingredients</u>

- 1 cup room-temperature coconut oil
- 1 cup almond butter

- 1/4 cup heavy whipping cream
- 10 drops liquid stevia
- Pinch sea salt

<u>Cooking Directions</u>
- Line the baking dish with material paper and put away.
- In a medium bowl, combine the salt, stevia, heavy cream, coconut oil, and almond butter until very smooth.
- Fill a baking dish with the mixture and smooth the top with a spatula.
- Refrigerate the dish until the fudge is firm, about 2 hours.
- Divide into 36 pieces and store for up to two weeks in a freezer-safe container.

Flourless chocolate cake fudge

<u>Ingredients</u>
- 1 cup (2 sticks) unsalted butter, plus additional butter for the pan
- 8 ounces chopped bittersweet chocolate
- 1 1/4 cups sugar
- 6 large eggs
- 1 teaspoon unadulterated almond extricate
- 1 c. unsweetened cocoa powdering
- Whipped cream, for serving

<u>Cooking Directions</u>
- Heat stove to 350°F. Lightly grease a 9-inch springform pan that has been lined with parchment.

- In a medium saucepan, melt the butter and chocolate together over medium heat, stirring frequently, until smooth.

- Let the mixture cool slightly for five minutes. Add sugar and blend to consolidate. After incorporating each egg one at a time, blend in the almond extract and cocoa powder until smooth.

- Pour the batter into the prepared pan and bake for 25 to 28 minutes or until the centre is just set. After cooling for ten minutes in the pan on a wire rack, remove the cake and allow it to cool completely.

- Dust with cocoa and present with whipped cream whenever wanted.

Coconut macaroons

<u>Ingredients</u>

- 1 14-ounce can of sweetened condensed milk 1 teaspoon 1/2 tsp. pure almond extract
- 1/4 cup almond flour
- kosher salt
- 14 oz. of sweetened flaked coconut
- 12 oz. bittersweet chocolate

<u>Cooking Directions</u>

- Whisk together the salt, almond extract, and condensed milk in a large bowl. Speed in almond flour until very much mixed. Mix in the coconut thoroughly to coat. Refrigerate for 1 1/2 hours, twice stirring.

- Heat the oven to 350°F. Use material paper to line two baking sheets. Spread the mixture out 1 inch apart on the prepared sheets using packed heaping tablespoons. After rotating the sheets on racks halfway through baking, bake for 15 to 16 minutes until golden brown around the edges. Allow the cookies to cool on wire racks.

- Melt the chocolate according to the package instructions once the cookies have cooled. Place on parchment paper or wax paper after dipping the bottoms in chocolate and letting the excess drip off. Drizzle the remaining chocolate over the tops after they have all been dipped and set.

Strawberry coconut crust cheesecake

<u>Ingredients</u>
- 4 large eggs divided
- 3/4 cup sugar divided
- 2 cups sweetened shredded coconut
- 1 lemon
- 3 8-ounce packages of room-temperature cream cheese; 3/4 cup sour cream
- 1 tablespoon
- 2 tsp. potato starch unadulterated vanilla concentrate
- 1 tbsp. strawberry jam,
- half a pound Small strawberries

<u>Cooking Directions</u>
- Preheat the oven to 375°F. Cover a 9-inch springform dish with cooking splash.

- Place the whites of two eggs in a medium bowl and the yolks in a small bowl. Whisk egg whites with 1 tablespoon sugar until frothy; add the coconut. Bake for 15 to 25 minutes, or until the mixture is evenly distributed on the pan's bottom and the centre is golden brown in spots and the edge is golden brown; let cool for 15 minutes. Lessen stove temperature to 325°F.
- In the meantime, zest and juice the lemon, obtaining approximately 2 teaspoons of zest and 3 tablespoons of juice, and set it aside. Beat cream cheese, sour cream, potato starch, vanilla, 3/4 cup sugar, 2 tablespoons lemon juice, and a large bowl with an electric mixer until smooth. Beat in the egg yolks that were left over and the remaining two eggs, one at a time. Bake for 35 to 40 minutes, or until the centre is still slightly wobbly and the edge is set. Refrigerate cheesecake for at least four hours to chill completely in the pan.
- Whisk together two tablespoons of sugar and the remaining tablespoon of lemon juice in a bowl while the cheesecake is chilling. Add berries and toss, then let sit for at least 15 minutes. Serve cheesecake with the reserved lemon zest.

Cocoa-nutty lime tart

<u>Ingredients</u>
- 3 tbsp. butter
- 3 ounces semisweet chocolate
- 3 cups of sweetened coconut shredded

- 1 brick (8 ounces) softened cream cheese
- 3 limes
- 1 can (14 ounces) for garnish

<u>Cooking Directions</u>
for sweetened condensed milk
- Preheat the oven to 325°F. Oil 9-inch tart container with removable base.
- Heat the butter and chocolate in a large microwave-safe bowl for 30 seconds at a time until just melted. Mix in the coconut. Press the mixture evenly into the pan's bottom and upside with your hands; position on a cookie sheet Bake for twenty minutes until firm. Completely cool.
- Beat cream cheese in a large bowl on high speed until smooth. Grate 1 teaspoon zest from limes and squeeze 1/2 cup juice; beat in condensed milk and cream cheese until smooth. Fill cooled covering; until set, chill for two hours. can be prepared one day in advance. Add lime zest and slices as a garnish.

www.ingramcontent.com/pod-product-compliance
Lightning Source LLC
Chambersburg PA
CBHW072246260726
48659CB00004BA/1373